The Drop Zone Diet

'This book will not only transform your weight, but your health too' Glynis Barber, actress and fitness instructor of *Glynis Barber's Anti-Aging Yoga Secrets* DVD

'Easy, simple and healthy food by a lady who loves to eat well. This book proves you can eat delicious, fresh food and still lose weight! What's not to love about this book!' Brian Turner CBE, chef and restaurateur

'The Drop Zone Diet transformed me into a fit, healthy bundle of energy – I loved it!' Aisleyne Hogen Wallace, presenter and model

The Drop Zone Diet

JEANNETTE JACKSON

MICHAEL JOSEPH
an imprint of
PENGUIN BOOKS

MICHAEL JOSEPH

Published by the Penguin Group
Penguin Books Ltd, 80 Strand, London WC2R ORL, England
Penguin Group (USA) Inc., 375 Hudson Street, New York, New York 10014, USA
Penguin Group (Canada), 90 Eglinton Avenue East, Suite 700, Toronto, Ontario, Canada M4P 2Y3
(a division of Pearson Penguin Canada Inc.)
Penguin Ireland, 25 St Stephen's Green, Dublin 2, Ireland (a division of Penguin Books Ltd)
Penguin Group (Australia), 707 Collins Street, Melbourne, Victoria 3008, Australia
(a division of Pearson Australia Group Pty Ltd)
Penguin Books India Pvt Ltd, 11 Community Centre, Panchsheel Park, New Delhi – 110 017, India
Penguin Group (NZ), 67 Apollo Drive, Rosedale, Auckland 0632, New Zealand
(a division of Pearson New Zealand Ltd)
Penguin Books (South Africa) (Pty) Ltd, Block D, Rosebank Office Park,
181 Jan Smuts Avenue, Parktown North, Gauteng 2193, South Africa

Penguin Books Ltd, Registered Offices: 80 Strand, London WC2R ORL, England

www.penguin.com

First published 2013
001

Extract o... ...ssion of

Set in 13.5/16pt Garamond MT Std
Typeset by Jouve (UK), Milton Keynes
Printed in Great Britain by Clays Ltd, St Ives plc

A CIP catalogue record for this book is available from the British Library

ISBN: 978–1–405–90933–4

www.greenpenguin.co.uk

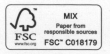

Penguin Books is committed to a sustainable
future for our business, our readers and our planet.
This book is made from Forest Stewardship
Council™ certified paper.

ALWAYS LEARNING   **PEARSON**

This book is dedicated to Sarah, my pride and joy.

Contents

PART THREE

Day 15 and Beyond

Foreword

The Drop Zone Diet is revolutionary in the field of health and weight loss as it is **100 per cent** based on pure health foods that offer true hope for the millions of people stuck in a negative cycle of powder/liquid dieting and junk food binge eating.

This book is written by my friend and colleague nutritional biochemist Jeannette Jackson and offers cutting-edge information on the science and genetics of weight gain; how you can positively affect *your own* health, despite a family predisposition to being overweight and unhealthy; and the scientific health benefits of the foods that you will eat on the diet.

Yet Jeannette also displays her personal experience as a woman and a mother, so the book is comforting and supportive in an emotional capacity too. It offers strategies to combat negative thought patterns and low self-esteem that can often be the difference between success and failure for so many women, and it explores emotional eating and how to learn to support yourself through challenging times.

In short, this book is a delight of wonderful, healthy foods, the healthiest weight-loss book around and a life-coach tool too!

Jeannette has gained vast experience through her travels across Europe, working with individuals and organizations, helping people and businesses to be healthy and well, and it shows in this book. She's heard every reason and excuse for not having the health and body you want, and she cuts through these to the truth; to once and for all get you to the body you so desire.

I know that her passion and enthusiasm has been the catalyst for major life changes in her clients' lives, and anyone who has had the pleasure to attend one of her seminars or a one-to-one consultation knows that her energy and vitality is infectious, and her drive to help others is more a vocation than a profession. She's a shining example that when you transform your energy, you cannot help but feel better, and in feeling better you reach further in your goals and dreams AND you have the energy to follow them through.

I also love that Jeannette shows her sense of humour when she entitles all the chapters in a similar way to her favourite TV programme, *Friends*.

So in true *Friends* style, this book (drum roll please . . .)

. . . Is the One Where You Transform Your Life!

I recommend this book to all who are ready for the purest of health and lifestyle transformations.

My advice is that you take the time to relish the colours and flavours of these dishes, and let the miracle of nature bring you back to where you belong.

Beautifully healthy, vibrant and well.

Jan de Vries
World-renowned Health Care Expert and author
of the By Appointment Only series of healthcare books.

Introduction

You thought you were simply buying a diet book – an extreme diet book that will help you to lose 14 pounds in 14 days. And you *have* bought a book that will do exactly that, but *The Drop Zone Diet* will also offer something quite different along-side. This book will help you to transform your health and wellbeing in the long term to such an extent that this will be the *last time* you ever have to diet again! You are now the proud owner of a 'triple-whammy' book that will help you to lose weight, feed your brain and boost your energy, all at the same time.

The Drop Zone Diet is an extreme diet for people who are in despair about their weight – who feel they have nowhere else to turn, and whose desire to lose weight quickly is making them feel panicky and anxious.

Physically . . . This diet is for people who, over the years, have taken drastic measures in a bid to shift excess weight. These include skipping meals, taking weight-loss tablets, or existing on just lettuce leaves or a single food type for days. The Drop Zone Diet is perfect for you if you tend to feel dizzy or lack concentration because you are so hungry; if you starve and then binge; if you are enticed by diets such as the 'water-only' diet, the 'tape-worm' diet or the 'cabbage-soup' diet, which promise instant results; or even if you try to shorten the day by going to bed early in order to reduce the number of hours during which you can be tempted by food!

Psychologically . . . This diet is for people who are ashamed of their bodies, embarrassed by being fat, and so dismayed when they go into a changing room that they leave the clothes store empty-handed.

Does this sound like you? Do you wear all-black or voluminous clothing to disguise your shape? Do you reject social invitations because you can't find anything to wear? Has your size contributed to feelings of depression and anxiety? If any of these scenarios apply to you, the Drop Zone Diet will provide the tools you need to get straight back on track and feeling good about yourself again.

Designed by a scientist and a leading UK chef, the Drop Zone Diet is not only satisfying and delicious, but it brings hope to millions of people who want to get their weight and health on a level playing field quickly and efficiently. You *can* lose up to 14 pounds in 14 days because this diet gives you the mental strength and confidence to stick to a plan and achieve results. Your improved confidence (not to mention your weight loss) will act as a springboard to put you back in charge of the food you eat, and as you start to look and feel the way you've always wanted, your confidence and self-esteem will soar, helping you to feel good about yourself. People who feel good about themselves look after themselves – a big part of that is eating healthily and well, and sustaining a healthy weight.

Whatever the reasons for your weight gain, there is a solution. Together, you and I will work out the things that have knocked you off track when you've dieted in the past. We'll explore why you climb back on the horse, only to fall off again; what *exactly* it is that causes you to fail over and over again. We'll look at your strengths and weaknesses, and establish how to align the two to ignite a passion and a desire so big that you'll power right through to your ultimate goal and lose all the weight you want. This time it's different. This time you *will* succeed.

Not a Crash Diet

The Drop Zone Diet is not a crash diet. By definition, crash diets cause the body to do just that: crash. They do not support the body's basic metabolic functions, leaving it depleted, lacking nutrients and exhausted. This is the reason for the chronic fatigue and cravings you will often experience when you choose to diet this way.

Metabolism is a process that takes place in all living organisms. It's rather like a complex production line on which literally thousands of chemical reactions take place within every single cell. These reactions keep our bodies functioning and alive. There are two types of metabolism that are worth knowing about. The first is 'catabolism', a process that breaks down the molecules from the food we eat (such as fats and sugars) into even smaller molecules that can be used to provide little units of energy when we need them. The second type of metabolism is 'anabolism', which then takes these little units of energy to build up our bodies (allowing us to grow taller, for example, or our bones to be made stronger).

In a nutshell, your metabolism converts food into energy that is then used by the body. In order to run smoothly, your hormones need to function properly, your blood sugar needs to be balanced, and macronutrients (fats, carbs and proteins) and micronutrients (vitamins and minerals, and other trace elements) need to be present in sufficient quantities. As simplistic as it may seem, our bodies need *food* in order to function, and for our metabolisms to do their job. Crash diets and slimming pills rob the body of the very basic things your metabolism needs. With no energy going in, there will be none coming out! You *will* feel exhausted on these diets; you *will* crave foods because your body is calling out for instant refuelling, and you *will* put on any weight you've lost straight after your diet because your body will be desperate to restock its energy supplies with full-fat foods and sugars. What's more, because you've been starving yourself, your metabolism will have slowed itself down, to make the most of what food there is on offer. It can take some time to readjust, so when you do start eating normally after a diet, your food isn't used as quickly or efficiently as it was before, causing more fat stores to be laid down.

Why This Diet is Different

The Drop Zone Diet is unique because it is nutritionally balanced. Every single food is chosen for its nutritional impact and its ability to boost your health, while working *with* your body to support smooth, easy weight loss. Underpinning the programme are supplements, which help to keep your energy levels steady and prevent cravings. These supplements also support your body between meals, when you may normally experience an energy dip (i.e., around 11am, 3pm and 8pm). We'll look at these a little later.

The Drop Zone Diet is effectively nutrition in motion. Even the soups are not just nourishing stand-alone meals, but a combination of energy-boosting carbohydrate superfoods and power proteins to build muscle and encourage beautiful skin and hair. The diet contains vibrant foods that are prepared and served in a natural state to enable you to achieve health and wellbeing on all levels. By feeding your body and brain everything it needs to function at optimum level, you will feel alert, energized and satisfied. Energy is manufactured via a chain of chemical reactions, and if you get the elements right you will experience a true alignment that will not only ensure the success of this diet, but allow you to get in touch with the thinner, inner you!

A Little About Me

I designed the Drop Zone Diet as a scientist. I wrote it as a woman.

Before embarking on a career as a scientist, I began my working life as an assistant in costume and make-up for theatre and television. I witnessed first hand the anxiety people experience when they are in view of others – especially in front of an audience or camera, but even sometimes just within a group. I was perplexed to see beautiful, hugely successful people suffering panic attacks in the privacy of their dressing rooms – wracked with insecurities about their looks, their bodies and everything else. I remember being transfixed when they were able to switch themselves 'on' to shine for the public. You'd never know that they were actually riddled with deep insecurities. In particular, I remember working with Ruby Wax. Her public persona is that of a brash, loud-mouthed American; in reality, she was nervous and almost shy off-camera. It has recently transpired that Ruby suffered from years of depression, and that doesn't surprise me. Trying to put on a face for the public is exhausting and demoralizing; eventually it all catches up with you.

Being privy to this backstage world helped me to understand the battle between 'private' and 'public' personae. Perhaps there is a 'you' who feels lost and insecure in the privacy of your own home, but paints on the lipstick and sucks it all in to go out into the world every day with a smile on your face. We do this because society dictates that this is the norm. What needs to change is how we feel about ourselves when we aren't playing the role of someone else, the 'public' you. A lot of my work helps people to become content and happy in their bodies, no matter what their size. Balancing our private and public selves and unifying them is a recipe for positive emotional health and, ultimately, the type of self-esteem that will drive you to look after yourself properly.

Having fulfilled my dream of working in television, I eventually decided to pursue my other main interest: nutrition. I went on to complete a two-year nutritional therapy course and began to help people establish healthy eating plans to boost health and wellbeing. I discovered that people came to me not just to lose weight and change their diets, but to get some emotional support as well. Years of poor nutrition had impacted upon their self-confidence and self-esteem to the point that many of them couldn't even remember feeling good about themselves. Behind closed doors, my clients didn't need to pretend any more, and they were able to open up about their insecurities and worries. With a little guidance, they were able to see the emotional impact that poor nutrition was having on their lives. Failing to provide the body with adequate fuel had not just caused problems with their weight, but it had affected their health on every level – including emotionally.

It quickly became obvious that many people knew *what* to eat (fresh fruit and vegetables, for example), but they gravitated towards unhealthy choices because their bodies craved sugar, fat, alcohol and any other number of quick-fix, instant-energy foods that caused their blood sugar to soar and then dip alarmingly, not to mention causing them to pile on weight. These types of diets left people tired, hungry, deflated and, in many cases, fat!

I was intrigued by the chemical changes within the body that drive us to eat the wrong foods, even when we do know how to eat well. I decided to go beneath the nutrition to the science, to better understand the role that food has on the brain and the body. I completed a three-year, full-time degree in biochemistry and the missing pieces of the puzzle fell into place. With the knowledge I gained, I could go further to help people, and that's when the Drop Zone Diet was born.

When designing this diet, I set out to create a supremely healthy, quick weight-loss diet that would offer all-day support to the body, thus preventing energy dips which often cause people to struggle and then succumb to cravings. I produced a diet that would be ideal for busy people who don't have time to cook elaborate meals, with quick, simple foods that would offer energy, health and, above all, weight loss in the easiest, most straightforward way possible.

At the outset, I passed the diet to existing clients who worked in television and the media, so that I could monitor the results. They were, quite honestly, staggering. I had a designed a formula that actually worked:

The world's healthiest foods

+

minimal calories

=

quick, easy weight loss

+

improved confidence and self-esteem

A Diet that Really Works

On this diet, there are no gimmicks, no food-combining, no calorie-counting, no classes to attend and no sponsors. The only thing required is for you to be passionate, prepped and ready to change your life with a little help from me and Mother Nature, who provides the most glorious foods.

Initially the Drop Zone Diet was designed for celebrities and models to use before a photo shoot, casting or filming, to help them drop weight rapidly whilst looking amazingly vibrant, fit and healthy. Many of these women were eating as little as possible in an attempt to lose weight quickly. However, the tiny quantities of food they were eating were so nutritionally poor, they were left feeling exhausted and depleted. Many gave in to night-time binges because their bodies were in desperate need of fuel. The truth is that these girls didn't look their best, because nutritious food is necessary to get that glow of good health.

As a biochemist, I knew that I could design a diet with a minimum of calories to help support quick weight loss, and I also knew how to make those calories work hard! Everything in the Drop Zone Diet has maximum nutritional impact, so that your body is being fed the most amazing superfoods as it lets go of old fats and toxins. The results spoke for themselves. People finished the diet looking vibrant and healthy, and feeling energized, fit and well. Best of all, they slept better, had clearer skin and were committed to eating well to continue experiencing the results!

The truth is that no advocate of healthy eating happily recommends a rapid weight-loss diet. I'd much rather encourage people to lose weight as part of a holistic, healthy lifestyle; however, there is a growing and insatiable desire within our society to do things instantly, no matter what the cost. People are becoming more and more desperate to lose weight, and some are taking very drastic action to get the bodies they want. I came to the conclusion that fighting this demand for instant results wasn't going to benefit anyone; people were going to continue to seek ways to drop pounds, regardless of the health implications. It seemed to me that it made much more sense to help people to achieve their goal in the healthiest way possible. Designing a rapid weight-loss diet based on nourishing meals would not only give me an opportunity to educate people about the benefits of wholesome food, but also show them that it is possible to eat nutritious food, lose weight and look and feel great throughout the process.

In my professional capacity as a scientist, I used my knowledge and skills to design a diet that cuts through the hype, fear and greed that currently underpins the weight-loss industry. I concentrated on factual, state-of-the-art research into the nutritional benefits of natural health foods, and their ability to work together to support weight loss in a simple, effective way. As a woman, I am a mother, a daughter, a friend, a colleague and a lover, and I care deeply about the health of those I love. I fear for my daughter in a world that celebrates a quest for celebrity-style emaciation. The near-skeletal female forms in some glossy magazines terrify me, and make me fearful for the future. By creating the Drop Zone Diet I hoped to re-educate the palates of my clients so that they would naturally veer towards healthy, life-giving foods when they were tired, stressed and busy, rather than turning to junk foods that caused the problems in the first place.

> ### Model mania
>
> I was recently working as a consultant for one of the world's leading sports brands, and one of the make-up artists told me that some models sent to Africa for assignments secretly hope to get chronic diarrhoea while there, to help them look thinner on the shoots!

Young women have gone to extreme lengths to achieve tiny sizes. The 'cotton-wool' diet is just one example. Yes, people do actually eat cotton wool to fill up their tummies. The lunacy is terrifying. I designed the Drop Zone Diet to help women (and men) lose weight quickly but sensibly, without risking their physical and emotional health in the process.

Diet Madness

The weight-loss industry has increased dramatically over the past two decades, with snack bars, drinks, powders, patches, sprays and all sorts of tablets and meals in packets now readily available. The manufacturers are savvy. They've done their research and know that we will probably do almost anything to get the body we want so much. We'll even overlook health risks if instant results can be achieved. They feed us up to thin us down again, all the while gorging on our insecurities.

No one wants to be caught in the 'ring of shame' in the glossy magazines. Unflattering 'zoomed-in' photographs of the physical flaws of people in the public eye are printed for readers to comment on and gossip about. Celebrities are so terrified of not having the perfect bodies they take drastic measures to stay thin (often too thin). Unfortunately many people then follow their lead.

We don't stand much of a chance when the giants of media and manufacturing work their magic in the supermarkets, even employing psychologists to help them defeat us. We know what we should be eating, but how can we avoid being tempted by products that are cannily packaged and advertised, and then placed directly at eye level when we scan the shelves? Within the supermarket we are a captive audience, often buying on impulse. The food industry is designed to take advantage of that!

Long-term weight loss relies upon sticking firmly to a goal and ignoring (as much as possible) the temptations around us. That's hard to do when we are hungry, tired and in need of instant energy and maybe even comfort, but it is possible to create change. By feeding your body healthy, natural food, you won't crave junk. You'll have stable energy levels throughout the day, so you won't end up shovelling in rubbish. The Drop Zone Diet has been created to do just that. You'll sleep peacefully and wake up refreshed and raring to go. This will feed your determination to succeed, and as you become happy and at peace with your shape, you'll actively seek out the foods that make you look and feel so fantastic.

Putting down the rope

When you begin a diet, do you find that you crave goodies more than ever? Do the advertisements seem brighter? Do the chocolates look more meltingly delicious, the bread smell yummier? It can seem like an endless battle to stay on the straight and narrow, but there is a solution. I call it 'putting down the rope'.

It is possible to end the struggle by making the decision not to engage in it any longer. Imagine yourself playing Tug of War against an opponent. The harder you pull, the harder they pull. But when you put down the rope, the game is over. The same goes for the war against overeating – or choosing the wrong foods. When you are really pulling (trying hard to be good), it somehow seems much harder.

I suggest you put down the rope now, which signifies that you are psychologically ready to proceed – you are ready for an adult relationship with food, ready to embrace the long-term impact of making good, nutritious choices. You are not denying yourself because you genuinely won't want or need unhealthy food any longer. If you can establish this frame of mind at the outset, you'll find that the temptations simply don't have the lure they once did. You aren't playing that game any more!

The long-term dieter

I never realized how bad I was feeling until I did the Drop Zone Diet. I knew I wanted to lose weight and was constantly on the search to find the holy grail of quick fixes. I have literally done every diet on the block.

And last year I felt a massive pressure to lose weight when my husband and I were invited on a company trip to Dubai with all the other sales reps and their partners. I really didn't want to be a white, beached whale next to some real beauties by the pool, so I went to some ridiculous extremes to lose weight. I bought slimming tablets and went to spas to get 'sucked' by hydrotherapy and other treatments. It cost me a fortune and didn't work. Stupid!

A colleague recommended the Drop Zone Diet and it transformed my life. I had forgotten how it feels to have energy. I was so tired all the time that I just got used to it. I used to try and crawl my way out of the 'tired pit' by existing on cakes and biscuits for energy, but that just made me heavier and more sluggish. Once I'd done the diet I had *real* energy – proper full-on bounceability – that meant I got home from work with plenty of energy to do things in the evening. The weight dropped off *easily*. This diet changed my life and my confidence has soared.

Ready to Go

I created the Drop Zone Diet for you and for every friend and client who has begged me to help them lose weight. This is an *extreme* diet, because I know that you want results – and fast. In fact, if there is one thing I've learned over the past couple of decades, it is that people need to see a shift almost immediately. If they don't see the desired outcome in a short space of time, they quickly move on to something else. We live in a quick-fix society and we're becoming increasingly used to getting what we need at the click of a mouse. Did you know that the average person spends just seven seconds on a website before deciding to click or move on? That's three blinks of an eye!

By ensuring that you see results – and by making the diet abundantly achievable – the Drop Zone Diet will take you off that merry-go-round of faddy, perpetual dieting. You can definitely lose up to 14 pounds in 14 days, on a diet that will feed the very core of you: your liver, your spleen, your brain, your skin and even your emotions! Your body will devour this diet, and positively sigh with relief that it is *finally* getting what it needs to function at optimum level.

I am deeply proud of this diet and the results it achieves. I've been picking up the pieces of the weight-loss industry for far too long now, and really want to offer something healthy and positive to help people make the changes they want towards happiness, health and balanced weight. It may be quick, but it's not a 'quick fix' because it changes the way you think about food in the long term. The Drop Zone Diet is a soothing balm in our barmy world!

I want to help you get back to 'you'. You are strong. You are tenacious and you have spirit. If someone you loved was in danger, you would roar like a lion and stand between him or her and a speeding truck. However, somewhere along the line you have forgotten to do this for yourself – forgotten how to protect yourself with the same vigour and determination, to care for yourself with the love that you offer to others, and to want the very best for yourself, just as you do for them.

Let's draw on that strength and spirit now. Are you telling me that you can continue to be defeated . . . by a doughnut? The time is right for change and you are ripe for good health. Let's get started, and enter the Drop Zone together.

PART ONE
Getting into the Zone

CHAPTER 1

The One Where We Put
First Things First

So why is the Drop Zone Diet different? Well, I believe it's because it is a *spiritual* diet. No, not *that* type of spiritual. I don't mean living on mung beans, wearing organza and growing long, flowing hair! According to the *Oxford English Dictionary*, the word 'spiritual' means 'closely akin in interests, attitude and outlook'. In terms of this diet, I suggest that success lies in becoming aligned with yourself emotionally and physically, creating a congruent, consistent 'you' who lives a life of colourful, vibrant continuity around food and nutrition. I'm sorry to tell you that you can't have it all. You can't be slim and then eat all the pies. The maths doesn't add up!

Getting yourself to a place where you really want to be – somewhere that every bit of you wants to be – will allow you to feel aligned. There is a power that comes from feeling this that will provide you with the desire, dedication and discipline to succeed.

You Have to Want It

I know you *want* to lose weight, so getting your desire up to scratch may not be a problem. Or is it? Sometimes you want it like you've never wanted anything before; sometimes, quite honestly, you can't be arsed. So how *much* do you want it?

A bit today, a lot tomorrow and desperately before you go on holiday? Are you pretty blasé on Friday nights, but completely focused on Monday mornings? Do you want it less on an average rainy afternoon than you do the day before the school reunion? #Just asking. There has to be consistency in your desire to drive yourself onwards or you will stay forever on that hamster wheel.

A quick question for you: Are you currently trying to lose *exactly* the same amount of weight you were at *exactly* the same time last year? If so, there is a clear pattern emerging. Why don't we work together to stabilize your weight so that you can simply get on with the business of enjoying your life?

If your desire is temporary, you'll get temporary results.

Always on a diet

According to industry analysts Mintel, one in four adults is on a diet at any one time in the UK. Some 37 per cent of those dieting are women, but 18 per cent of men are looking to lose weight, too.

When you desire change because you want *change*, and you want it above and beyond merely being thin, slim and gorgeous, then you *will* create change in the fundamentals in your life: there will be no going back.

The beauty of the Drop Zone Diet is that you'll become more in tune with your body. You'll enjoy feeling fantastic so much that you'll continue to eat amazing foods even after the diet has finished. This is a *positive* cycle that produces both the end result you want (weight loss) as well as a life free from boring diets. If you are feeling fresh and lively, you are much more likely to reach for foods that encourage that feeling to continue. Like attracts like! In my opinion, when you feel heavy, congested and stuck, you end up craving foods that match that feeling, and you stay stuck in a rut. The Drop Zone Diet is all about vitality and freshness – eating foods with a life force to nurture and uplift you.

Dedication Matters

How dedicated are you to fulfilling your goal? It may be necessary to do work on eradicating some of the negative elements of your life and replacing them with something more positive. For example, if you spend time slagging yourself off for being fat, lazy, invisible (or too visible), useless or ugly, you'll need a significant mind shift.

Take a look at the following mindset questions devised by Martin Robert Hall, a sports performance expert and author of *Optimize Yourself.* He works with leading sportspeople, pushing them to achieve their dreams and goals in spite of their fears and insecurities.

1. How would you rate your attitude in life on a scale of 1–10, with 10 being the best it could possibly be?
   1 2 3 4 5 6 7 8 9 10

2. How clear are you about what goals you would like to achieve in the next six months, and how persistent are you in terms of achieving your goals? Score 10 for very clear.
   1 2 3 4 5 6 7 8 9 10

3. How optimistic are you that you will achieve the body you want, with 10 being the most optimistic?
1 2 3 4 5 6 7 8 9 10

4. How would you rate your patience (with 10 being most patient)? Are you committed to making small and consistent improvements or do you become frustrated when you don't see instant miracles?
1 2 3 4 5 6 7 8 9 10

5. How enthusiastic are you about starting the Drop Zone Diet and enjoying the results (with 10 being incredibly enthusiastic)?
1 2 3 4 5 6 7 8 9 10

6. In general, how would you rate your level of self-discipline (with 10 being most disciplined)?
1 2 3 4 5 6 7 8 9 10

7. How clear are you about what you want to achieve in your lifetime, with 10 being crystal clear?
1 2 3 4 5 6 7 8 9 10

8. How would you rate your mindset in terms of being free of fear and self-doubt? 10 is unaffected and 1 is constantly slowed down on a daily basis.
1 2 3 4 5 6 7 8 9 10

9. How would you rate your ability to operate outside your comfort zone? Do you stretch yourself con-

stantly (10) or are you confined to living in your comfort zone, avoiding everything that makes you feel uncomfortable (1)?

1 2 3 4 5 6 7 8 9 10

Gauging the results

To experience the benefits and wonderful transformative effects of the Drop Zone Diet, you'll need to get yourself into a position where you can confidently score at least '8' for each of these questions. I need you to be buzzing about this exciting opportunity and thrilled about carrying a beautiful, fit, healthy body around with you after the diet has finished. The Drop Zone Diet is about transformation, and the more deeply you can embed your determination, excitement and persistence throughout the diet, the greater the rewards – and the longer lasting they will be. Over the 14 days of the Drop Zone Diet, you'll have to believe that nothing is as important as feeling good. A positive mantra is crucial. If you scored below '5' on some of the questions above, it's worth working hard to establish the right frame of mind before you begin – you need to really believe that anything is possible and that the Drop Zone Diet is going to be the catalyst for change that will charge up your life, push you straight out of your comfort zone and give you the determination and motivation to set and maintain goals in the sunny new future that now shines ahead of you. Being passionate about change and the process of change will drive your success. Just *believe*! By the end of the diet I can guarantee you'll be scoring all 10s!

Youthful joy

I recently visited a nursery as part of my research and interviewed a group of four-year-old children. I asked them how they felt when they woke up in the morning. The answer from almost every child was: happy, hungry, playful and in love with Mummy!

I then interviewed a group of middle-aged women and asked them the same question. Invariably they replied: exhausted, fat, shattered, depressed, tired and stressed.

So, what happens in the intervening years to take us from happy, excited, positive children to stressed, exhausted adults? And how can we get back to our childlike selves?

It's a female thing

Let's be honest: you eye up other women, don't you? Women eye up other women: their shoes, clothes, handbags and hair. In fact, women often eye up other women more than they do men! Not in a sexual way, but as a point of comparison. Is she thinner or fatter than me? Happier than me? We make snap decisions about other women based on their appearance and both consciously and unconsciously relate our own happiness quota in life to theirs. The childminder who looked after my daughter when she was a baby once told me that my life is easier than hers and full of more happiness because I am slim and she is fat! We assume that when other people have what we desire, they also have the happiness we crave.

A recent study by Incognito found that the first thing women notice about other women is how fat or thin they are in relation to themselves. Two thousand women aged between 18 and 45 were asked how they form first impressions, and the results say a lot about us! In order, we notice:

1. Weight
2. Foundation (are they wearing too much?)
3. Dress sense
4. Hairstyle
5. Smile
6. Skin (including spots)
7. Height
8. Visible hair roots
9. Level of fake tan
10. Eye make-up

So if we spend a good deal of our time comparing ourselves to others, what are we doing to our self-worth? We put ourselves down and raise others up. This is probably one of the most negative activities that we regularly undertake, and it's time to switch that to something more positive. To reinforce your confidence and self-esteem in the long term, you need to be kind to yourself, cut yourself some slack and *stop* comparing your 'inner' world with the 'outer' world of others! To enjoy this diet and achieve optimum results, you need to take care of yourself. This directly affects your self-worth and helps you to feel good about yourself.

Remember that when we look at other people, we see the image that they *choose* to project to the world! We are effectively getting an edited version of who they really are. Scratch below the surface of most people (myself included!) and you'll find insecurities and fears. The difference is that some people allow these fears to overwhelm them, leading to a life of submission and inertia, while others acknowledge these feelings and then put them to one side in order to live a life of health and happiness on many levels. You can be in the second group! And the good feelings that you'll experience as your confidence grows and your self-esteem increases will be a catalyst for positive change. You can actively say no to habits and patterns around food and nutrition that no longer serve you, and start to live your life with optimism, positivity and vigour!

The PR girl

> Working in public relations made it so difficult for me to lose weight. It's an incredibly social world and part of the job involves taking clients out for meals; and if you're not entertaining, then you're off to the bar after work. There's quite a lot of pressure to do this, or you are not seen as a 'team player'. To make matters worse, I'm naturally on the large side and PR is full of slim young things who are all full of confidence. My self-esteem took a battering! After trying a million different diets I became exhausted, and I was sick to death of calorie- or point-counting. By the time I heard about the Drop Zone Diet I'd got to the stage where I was skipping meals to 'save up' calories for later in the day – or even later in the week! I was having major energy dips because of the lack of food. At one point, I seriously thought I had narcolepsy, as I just couldn't

keep my eyes open by mid-afternoon. The Drop Zone
Diet was a breath of fresh air in my life in so many
ways. It was easy, quick and delicious and it totally did
what it said on the tin. In the past I've lost weight but
felt miserable, moody, tearful and snappy (I realize
now that this was due to lack of vitamins from the
poor-quality diets). The Drop Zone Diet was different.
I honestly felt amazing right from the start and by the
end it looked like I'd been to a health farm! My skin
and hair were smooth and shiny, and my confidence
really did get the boost it needed.

Just being

How dedicated are you to creating the life you want? How do
you incorporate your dedication to yourself in the way you
act, think and perform each day? Do you function on autopilot and live most days like *Groundhog Day*? I once went to a
wonderful Buddhist retreat where part of the morning medi-
tation involved learning to practise 'being', which enhanced
dedication to living a healthy life. This practice would help to
sustain the Buddhists through the day. They would say things
like: 'Today I shall practise compassion', 'Today I shall practise peace' or 'Today I shall practise stillness'. For the
remainder of the day, they would be mindful of the mental
and emotional state they wanted to achieve. It is a skill that
I have taken away with me, and recommend to others.

How are you feeling?

How has your dedication to your life manifested itself?
How often do you feel regularly fulfilled? How do you feel
on a daily basis? Stressed, exhausted, time-poor, anxious,

depressed, agitated, irritable or moody? Take a look at the following quiz, and we'll get to the bottom of it all.

When the alarm clock goes off I . . .
a) Feel utterly exhausted
b) Snooze it until the last minute
c) Get up happily and feel awake and alert

By mid-morning I . . .
a) Feel the need for a snooze again
b) Need a sugar boost to keep me going
c) Have loads of energy and am still raring to go

At lunchtime I . . .
a) Grab a sandwich and eat at my desk
b) Forget what time it is and work until I am ravenous in the late afternoon
c) Take time away from my desk to eat a nutritious lunch

By mid-afternoon I . . .
a) Am always starving and snack on junk
b) Have an energy dip and need a quick fix of caffeine, sugar or nicotine
c) Eat fruit and healthy snacks to stave off natural hunger pangs

After work I . . .
a) Am so exhausted I need a drink to wind down
b) Go home to my family snappy and moody if I've had a bad day
c) Cook a replenishing dinner from scratch and enjoy winding down with family/friends

At bedtime I . . .
a) Feel stressed or agitated because I can't 'switch off'
   and fall asleep
b) Fall asleep exhausted but wake in the night worrying
   about work/problems
c) Relax and unwind by reading before bed and fall
   into restful sleep

It goes without saying that the 'c' answers are those that are best for your mind and your body. It is a 'c' lifestyle that we should all aim to achieve in order to live a healthy, balanced and peaceful life. Is it any wonder that many people fail to establish and stick to positive weight-loss goals when they are running around on empty – knackered, stressed and always trying to catch up?

To fully embrace this diet and remain focused, it's best to adopt a peaceful, contented approach to whatever life throws at you. Actions are effectively thoughts in motion, so if you choose a positive frame of mind, it will serve you well when the going gets tough. That's part of the dedication to weight loss and, most importantly, to you.

When you wake up in the morning, why not spend a few minutes remembering the Buddhist practice of being mindful? Select a word that sums up who you are when you're at your most contented. For the next 14 days, begin each day by saying 'Today I shall practise xxx'. I often like to use the word 'fluidity' because it implies going with the flow and yielding to what life has to offer each day. That doesn't mean 'succumbing', but going about my day with my principles intact, living my own life while others live theirs. If you set yourself a mindful task in this way, if you do waiver or get knocked off kilter emotionally, you'll know where to return in order to find alignment. The word fluidity is perfect to keep you positive as it implies movement, flow and energy. In fact, the Drop Zone Diet is all about fluidity. It's the difference between clear onion soup and thick, stodgy rice pudding. One moves effortlessly and flows beautifully with ease; the other is thick, heavy and congealing.

The importance of changing your mindset can't be under-estimated. Putting yourself in a place where you are able to experience positive emotions whilst weathering temptations and negative influences is essential. But you must also change your default setting! You may set out in a positive mindset, shifting from heavily processed and manufactured foods to fresh, real, 'alive' foods, but what happens when you become stressed and tired? At this point you will need to get your brain and your body to gravitate towards healthy foods for comfort and support. Dedicating yourself to this diet and to yourself will help you to begin to achieve this.

The mum

> I have three children between the ages of two and 17 (yes, the latest addition to the family was a lovely surprise), and I was not only sick of being fat but also very tired of being tired! I dragged my body out of bed every morning and then threw myself back into it every night in a state of utter exhaustion. I have a fantastic family and a lovely life but my tiredness was getting me down and I knew somehow it was connected to what I was eating. When I did the Drop Zone Diet I was transformed! Who knew that avocado on rice cakes could be so yummy? It was easy to follow and the food was delicious. I did it,

committed to it and I've reaped the results by losing a
stone. Much more importantly, however, my energy
has *rocketed*!

Creating Long-term Change

In order to instigate long-term change, you need to remove
chaos from your life and look at what you are 'constantly
doing' to create positive change. For too many people, the
only 'constant' is flitting from diet to diet, chasing a seemingly elusive body without success. Are your dietary patterns
and eating habits chaotic and inconsistent? Do you eat
healthy food on a good day but succumb to junk when you
are stressed, tired or hormonal?

I see many different types of dieters in my clinic and my
social circle, from yo-yo-dieters, to comfort eaters, to desperate-
measures dieters who starve themselves and then instantly
regain weight. However, many of us fall into two main cate-
gories: Monday-morning dieters and Kitchen-cupboard
dieters. Which one are you?

The Monday-morning dieter

You . . .

1. Decide every Sunday night that tomorrow is it!
   Tomorrow is definitely the first day of the rest of
   your wonderful skinny life.

2. Go to sleep feeling content that finally you are going
   to get the body that you want.

3. Wake on Monday morning full of promise.

4. Arrive at work with lots of fruit, water, salad and crispbreads in your bag.

5. Decline offers to meet friends for lunch, to avoid temptation.

6. Doggedly stick to your boring salad at lunchtime (feeling a bit left out) as everyone else eats delicious food from the deli.

7. Begin to flag around 3pm. (Maybe a quick Starbucks wouldn't hurt?)

8. Engage in a mental dialogue around 5pm, which goes something like this: 'Which biscuits, crisps or sweets have the fewest calories? Surely there must be something that contains chocolate, yet has zero calories?'

9. Decide by 5:10pm that you need to eat something or you'll faint. Reassure yourself that you are doing yourself a favour by having one teeny, tiny treat.

10. Arrive home exhausted to a low-fat, low-calorie microwave meal that is as appealing as the sole of a shoe.

11. Tuesday: repeat stages 4 to 10.

12. Wednesday: Pizza Hut. Resolve to start again on Monday.

The Kitchen-cupboard dieter

You . . .

1. Open the kitchen cupboards to confirm there's too much temptation in the house.

2. Decide to empty the cupboards and fridge of all biscuits, sweets, crisps and cakes.

3. Go to the supermarket and spend a fortune on fresh fruit and vegetables.

4. Go home, unpack bags, place fruit and vegetables in fridge and fruit bowl, which you place in a prominent position to remember to eat it.

5. Decide (just for tonight!) to have a takeaway, as there is no 'comfort food' in the house and it's been a tough day. Tomorrow you'll start on the fruit and vegetables.

6. Throw away old rotten fruit and vegetables ten days later and restock cupboards with biscuits, sweets, crisps and cakes because guests are expected.

7. Repeat cycle twice a month.

Do you recognize yourself? When it's spelled out like this, do you feel a little sheepish? Getting rid of the excuses and understanding the patterns that are undermining your progress towards a healthy weight and lifestyle can help you to conquer them.

Why Lose Weight?

It's fairly obvious that 99 per cent of us go on a diet to lose weight. We want to lose weight to look better because we believe that when we look better we will *feel* better! Ultimately, feeling good is what it's all about – feeling good is the holy grail that everyone is chasing: 'When I lose weight I will feel confident and happy and relaxed about my appearance.' But is that the reality?

Do you have any idea how many 'thin' women have been to see me in my private clinic, reporting feelings of exhaustion, depression, stress, anxiety and being run down? They may be thin, but they are ill and desperately unhappy too. Is that *really* the holy grail to which you are aspiring? The real nirvana has got to be looking fantastic *and* feeling amazing as well, hasn't it?

The Drop Zone Diet is designed to get you on track to do just that, by providing your body with the nutrients it needs for overall good health and wellbeing but few enough calories to get that excess weight off once and for all. When you start to look good, you'll start to think and feel better, too! When we feel good, our brain engages in the process of manufacturing positive neurotransmitters, which boosts your mood and levels of contentment even further. The whole process is utterly captivating and delicious!

If we adopt the Buddhist philosophy that we must 'go beneath the drama to the truth', we will find that the overwhelming reason for losing weight is to feel good about ourselves. We want to be happy. Try to remember that being skinny by itself isn't necessarily going to achieve that. What will achieve it is mindful eating, feeding your body living, energy-boosting, healthy foods that serve to balance and sustain you on all levels. The end result of this type of living is health and happiness and, of course, a balanced weight. You'll look and feel better than ever before because you are living your life in a positive way. You are doing what you are doing for *you*.

There is a lovely little allegory that appears in Stephen Covey's *7 Habits of Highly Effective People*. It's called 'The Professor and the Fish Tank'.

One day, while trying to help his students prioritize their studies and their free time, a professor placed a large, oblong fish tank on his desk and filled it with five large stones. He filled it until no more stones could fit in, and then he asked his students: 'Is the tank full?'

When they nodded, he pulled out a bag of small pebbles and poured them between the gaps of the large stones. When no more pebbles could be fitted in and around the big stones, he asked his students again, 'Is the tank full?'

When they nodded a second time, he pulled out a bag of sand and duly sifted it into all the tiny gaps between the stones and the pebbles. When no more sand would fit into the tank, he asked his students, 'Is the tank full?'

Once again, they agreed that it was. This time the professor pulled out a jug of water and poured it over the sand until it soaked it completely and reached the top of the tank. This time the tank really was full.

The professor said, 'We have to put the big things in our life first, and then we can fit everything else around that.'

I think that's a great way to remind us what is important in our lives and how it can get filled up with incidentals and trivialities that simply don't matter in the long run. So what are the big things in your life? What would be your stones? Family? Health? Career? Friends?

Stephen Covey proves that when you concentrate on the priorities in your life, happiness becomes second nature. People who do this naturally exude energy and vitality because they are living the life they love. So to enable us to get you the body that you would love to live in, we need to put first things first and find you some energy from which you can launch your desires. The Drop Zone Diet may be short, but its effects can last a lifetime. It will give you the energy to stick with your goals and transform your weight, and become a catalyst to create a positive and powerful shift in your life in general.

CHAPTER 2

The One Where We Get You Some Rocket Fuel

Your energy levels define your ability to live life to the fullest and achieve your goals. When you feel exhausted and shattered, it's almost impossible to stick to self-imposed limits, no matter how determined you may be. It's fine and dandy setting yourself targets, but when you've had a tough day at work, how can you be sure that you'll hit them? Have you in the past? Lack of energy and poorly considered goals can lead you straight into the 'inertia/apathy trap', and that's when things start to fall apart.

'I always have fantastic intentions when I get in the car to drive home from work and yet, by the time I've arrived at my front door, I've talked myself out of going to the gym, and invariably picked up a takeaway as a reward for working so hard all day. Good intentions gone right out of the window again!'

Inertia is effectively a mass (in this case, that's you – sorry!) that resists change in motion. It can also mean sluggishness and inactivity. In chemistry an inert gas has no catalytic capabilities. In other words, it lacks *oomph*! So how is *your* oomph? I bet you don't have much. Has your get-up-and-go got up and left?

I developed the phrase 'inertia/apathy trap' after I watched people going round and round in circles, stuck in a cycle of wanting or needing to lose weight but feeling overwhelmed. Their goal seemed like such a huge mountain to climb that they simply sat at the bottom of it in a state of inertia, trying half-heartedly or giving up altogether. The inertia/apathy trap can occur when your goals are ambiguous and poorly defined and the desire to follow them is weak. A classic example of this is: 'I want to lose weight but I'll wait until the very last minute before my holidays, and then panic!'

To achieve the results you want, a shift in motion (habits and patterns) will be necessary. This requires action and energy. You'll have to work out where and when you tend to lose momentum and determination, and develop strategies to get you through those periods. For example, if you always succumb to a takeaway after work, try having a small, healthy snack before you leave the office, or take a different route home. If you lack energy to hit the gym in the evenings, try to schedule your workout for the times when you feel most energetic.

There is a strange sort of schizophrenia that many of us experience when it comes to losing weight and even healthy eating. One part of the brain is saying, 'Right, healthy dinner of fresh fish and salad this evening' and the other (possibly louder) part of the brain says, 'But you've worked so hard . . . why not do the healthy thing tomorrow and enjoy a well-deserved takeaway and bottle of wine tonight?' The problem is that tomorrow never really comes! So how do we create a change in our mindset (and silence that devilish voice) to break the pattern?

Excuses, Moi?

I think I have heard literally every excuse in the book. You can't kid a kidder! Why can't you stick to a goal to lose weight and stay healthy? Do any of the reasons in the list below sound familiar? Tick off how many have interfered with your ability to achieve your weight-loss goals in the past.

1. I have to travel with my job so I can't stick to a healthy-eating routine
2. My partner isn't on a diet so I'm cooking different food for each of us
3. I crave sugary, sweet foods
4. I can manage the diet but I can't give up alcohol
5. I want to be able to socialize with my friends
6. I pick at the kids' meals
7. I have to attend breakfast/lunch meetings at work and they serve stodgy foods
8. We always have cakes and sweets in the office and it's hard to resist
9. I get stressed and shattered and need warm comforting food
10. I don't have time to prepare healthy food and smoothies all the time
11. I'm a rubbish cook
12. It's too expensive to buy healthy food
13. I don't like vegetables
14. I don't like salads
15. I don't like cold foods
16. I work irregular hours so it's difficult to get into a routine

17. I work shifts so I sleep most of the day
18. I'm so busy that I don't always get a lunch hour, and tend to eat anything to hand because I get so hungry later
19. I tend to graze and never really get hungry enough for a proper meal
20. I have low blood sugar, so I need to eat regularly
21. I have to pass McDonalds on way to/from work and lose my willpower
22. I don't do the cooking in our house, so it's difficult to regulate my diet
23. I work long hours and don't feel like cooking when I get in
24. I have no willpower
25. I have no spare time between my family commitments and work, etc.
26. Salads and vegetables are boring
27. I have an active social life and always eat out
28. I try, but I just can't stick to a diet
29. Every Monday morning I begin a diet and by Wednesday I've failed
30. There is too much temptation everywhere

1–5 Ticks

It should be relatively easy for you to stick to a diet in the short term, as you have a strong desire. Pick a time when you have a quiet social diary and let nothing get in the way of your quest to lose the excess weight. Practise some of the 'mindfulness' exercises in the previous chapter so that you are constantly reminded of your goal. Let nothing deter you from your path, and you will succeed. Your desire clearly outweighs the number of excuses you have to give up! You have positivity on your side and, with this, you can conquer anything!

5–10 Ticks

You are going to have to dig deep in order to achieve your goals in the long term; however, that doesn't mean you can't do it. You have to redefine some of your beliefs about healthy eating and get organized! Actively change your shopping habits and routines, and try to cook healthy meals in advance and freeze them (or think about buying a slow-cooker). Enlist the help of your best friends and get a 'healthy buddy' system going to keep each other motivated. Talk to your loved ones about how important this is for you, and enlist their support as well. To break the endless cycle of starting a diet with determination and then falling at the first hurdle, you'll need to flip every single excuse on its head. The Drop Zone Diet will do most of the work for you by giving you the energy you need to stick to your goals, but you need to be organized enough to make it easy to stay with it.

10+ Ticks

It's time to re-establish your priorities and make sure your health and wellness stay right at the top of the list. Either you have an extremely full and busy life and time is at a premium, or perhaps you have *too much* time on your hands, and you are bored by the monotony of daily life. Either way, something has to give and you'll need to be truthful with yourself. If you are madly busy and dashing around all the time, sit quietly for a while and establish where you exert all of your energy – and with whom. Drop the things in your life that aren't bringing you pleasure or improving your life (or the lives of your family) to any real extent. Try to get super-organized so that your routine is streamlined; for example, prepare break-fast and lunch for tomorrow the night before; meet a friend at the gym instead of at a restaurant; and get some more sleep and fit in a little exercise – I can't tell you how much more energetic you'll feel, even if it seems impossible now. A life spent catching up is exhausting because you are effect-ively chasing your own tail! Getting organized puts you in the driving seat of your life, and this is a place where you'll feel comfortable and proud to be.

And what if it's the opposite, and you are bored? I have to ask you: How can you be bored when the world is so abun-dant and vibrant? If your life has become too routine and you feel like you are experiencing the same things over and over again, it's worth establishing why you've let this happen. Do you crave stability, order, comfort and familiarity? There is nothing wrong with good, regular routines that provide structure to your life, but if things become too repetitive it becomes impossible to make changes or even see the poten-tial for change. You may need help to escape this rut, and to get your self-esteem and confidence back. Why not invest a little money in your future and hire a life coach? A profes-sional can help you to get back on track and see the bigger picture; he or she can help you to see a path to your goals, even if it seems impossible to imagine. In seminars I ask people how long they have been unhappy with their weight (or health or body), and many have felt this way for 10 years! If it seems like an extravagance to pay for help to get you back on track, consider this: the chances are you already pay professionals for things you can't do yourself; you pay the dentist or the hairdresser or the mechanic. Why not invest in yourself and your future? With someone to guide you, your excuses will fall away like autumn leaves.

Once you've faced up to your excuses, no matter what they are, you will be one step closer to achieving the weight and the lifestyle you want.

Try to remember, too, to remain mindful of how you operate from day to day. If you work on autopilot and order a large muffin and a cappuccino every morning, or automatically reach for the same foods at the supermarket every week, you'll need to stop and think. Bad habits are hard to break, but once you become aware of them, you'll be less likely to sabotage your efforts unconsciously. Actively set out to create new, healthier habits by questioning everything you eat, drink and do for the coming days. It's easier than you may think!

Finding Energy to Create More Energy

This may sound like a strange suggestion, but the truth is that you need to feel energetic in order to stick to your goals, get through rough patches and break the habits that always set you back. The Drop Zone Diet is not only an amazing way to kick-start the weight-loss process quickly and efficiently, but it also fills you with incredible energy that will drive the changes you want to make. We need to get your 'mass' in motion and get you actively involved in your own health revolution.

Let's start by working out how much effort you are prepared to put in to get the body you want. There is no doubt that the Drop Zone Diet will be the simplest weight-loss diet you've ever followed, but to achieve optimum results you need to change your eating habits in the long term. Many people claim to want to make changes, but then crack at the least resistance. They tend to think: What is the maximum gain I can get for the least effort? What about you? How much longer are you willing to be a quick-fix junkie? I asked 100 people the questions below, and wasn't surprised by the results. Most people said that while they would *prefer* to experience the life outlined in column A, in reality they would probably opt for column B because they are too stressed, tired, busy or time-poor to create consistent change in their lives. Take a look at the questions and see what you think.

A I am happy to . . .	B I would rather . . .
Learn how to cook healthy nutritious foods from scratch	Have food placed in front of me, ready prepared, whether that be a meal delivered by a nutritionist, a takeaway or a microwave ready meal
Prepare healthy snacks that I can take with me for healthy energy boosters	Go to Starbucks for a latte and cake
Take time to write a shopping list designed around foods that 'suit' my body and make me feel good	Use shakes/powders/slimming tablets if they will produce the right results
Go to the gym on a regular basis	Have liposuction
Learn meditation and relaxation techniques to use to unwind after work	Open a bottle of wine after work to unwind
Get up nice and early at the weekend and get into the country for some fresh air and exercise	Have a lie-in

If your answers mainly fall in column B, the chances are that you feel that you lack the energy to live a column-A lifestyle. The Drop Zone Diet will give you the energy you require to spend more of your time in column A. I'm positive that once you begin to live your life in this way, you'll want to stay there permanently. Using a biochemically designed diet plan, with key nutrients and supplements to boost energy, the Drop Zone Diet will prepare you physically to make changes long term.

The Drop Zone Diet – an injection of rocket fuel!

My electric toothbrush has a little window at the side with an indicator that tells me when the battery is getting low and needs recharging. Wouldn't it be great to have an indicator like this on our bodies? What would your energy levels be right now? Are you at 100 per cent charged and raring to go? Or are you significantly lower than that? Some people in my seminars admit to feeling like they are operating at about 20 per cent most of the time. That's no way to live your life and, quite frankly, it's no *wonder* you lack the determination and drive to stick to your goals.

> 'I feel like I have low-level jet lag most of the time. Stress affects my sleep, so I wake up tired. I end up grazing all day to keep myself going, and drink too much coffee and eat too many sugary foods to try to keep my blood-sugar levels up. No wonder I can't sleep. My brain is still fizzing!'

Do you need recharging? If so, where is this rocket fuel going to come from? How are we going to get your energy indicator up to the max? From the foods that you eat, that's how. Unlike plants, we humans can't get our energy from the sun. We can, however, *eat* those plants and get our energy that way!

All food groups are required for a healthy body. Proteins, carbs and fats all play a significant role in functional nutrition – in other words, foods that your body requires to perform at optimum level. Removing any one of these food groups long term is a big mistake, because all are necessary for overall health and wellbeing. All are necessary for *energy*. The recent craze for low- and even no-carbohydrate diets meant that huge swathes of the population began to live almost exclusively on fats and proteins. Not surprisingly, this fad has largely bombed and there is increasing evidence that not only does any weight lost on this type of diet pile back on as soon as normal eating habits are resumed, but overall health (in particular heart health) suffers, too. What's more, a diet that is too high in protein can put huge strain on the kidneys, which must excrete the excess nitrogen that a high-protein diet creates. In extreme cases, kidney disease can result.

Protein *is* important, and in the Drop Zone Diet you'll find both animal and vegetable forms to provide you with the amino acids you need to look and feel great. You'll also find carbohydrates, which are effectively 'energy' foods – but not the refined kinds of carbs! Likewise, natural sugars such as fruit and honey are definitely on the menu, but you won't experience those crazy 'sugar shock' moments where your body goes into overdrive and then crashes a little later. The truth is that when your body is nutritionally balanced, natural sugars found in fruit (and even in vegetables) will not negatively impact on either your blood sugar *or* your energy levels. You'll also be taking the mineral chromium, in supplement form, which helps to keep blood sugar steady (and reduce cravings); see page 122.

The Drop Zone Diet may be low in calories, but it is high in *all* of the key nutrients that your body needs for balance. You may wonder how you can feel energetic on so few calories, but the calories in this diet work *hard*. The foods you'll be eating are nutrient dense, and designed to boost energy on all levels.

Give me sunshine!

Eric and Ernie were very wise (pun intended) when they sang 'Bring Me Sunshine'. Without the sun, we would become seriously ill. We need the ultra-violet rays it provides to manufacture vitamin D, which not only protects against depression and insomnia, but also helps to manufacture a hormone known as calcitriol, which we need to extract calcium from our diet. I recommend getting outside in the sunshine – ideally for a brisk walk – for at least 15 minutes each day, to help you get the most from the sun.

And there is more. For metabolism to take place (in other words, for energy to be extracted from our food and used efficiently by the body), we need something called ATP (adenosine triphosphate), which is manufactured through a series of energy transfers and found cellular organelles called mitochondria in our cells. The more ATP there is in your body, the more energy you'll have. One way to ensure good levels of ATP is to ensure that you have plenty of B-complex vitamins in your body – in particular, vitamin B1 (thiamine). B vitamins are found in whole grains, pulses, yeast extract, asparagus, animal products, broccoli, bananas, potatoes, milk, yoghurt, nuts and fish. The Drop Zone Diet is jam-packed with B vitamins, which is just one of the reasons why your energy levels will rocket. Other supplements on the diet (such as Coenzyme Q10) will also help both during the diet and beyond (see pages 122–6).

Poor diet, stress, inadequate (or poor quality) sleep, an underactive thyroid gland and even an over-reactive immune system can all affect the way our bodies produce ATP and use it. The good news is that the Drop Zone Diet will not only create nutritional balance to help overcome this, but also encourage healthy sleep and relaxation. Furthermore, the foods the diet contains are easy to digest, reducing pressure on your digestive system and supporting energy production by feeding your body the right fats, carbs and proteins at the appropriate cellular levels to repair burnt-out adrenal glands caused by repetitive stress. You'll feel totally refreshed, boosted and raring to go!

So, we've got your energy levels sorted. We've worked out the best ways to overcome the excuses that tend to set us back. We're starting to think about the habits we've developed that cause us to overeat – even subconsciously. But what is a dieter's worst nightmare and biggest downfall? Cravings! Your mouth waters and your senses are on high alert for specific foods; even the strongest will in the world won't stop you from succumbing. How can the Drop Zone Diet keep you going? Let's find out.

CHAPTER 3

The One Where We Combat Cravings

Your IQ (intelligence quotient) is a score that reflects, not surprisingly, your intelligence. I've worked on a one-to-one basis with clients for over 20 years, and I know what an intelligent (and sometimes devious) bunch you are! In my work, I came up with the term 'EQ', your 'eating quotient'. It's not just a play on words. I use this term with my clients when we look at the intelligent and often elaborate schemes they've devised to feed their cravings and their unhealthy eating habits. Cravings can overcome even the strongest willpower and undermine the best planned goals. They are the result of a combination of factors, including blood-sugar levels, nutritional deficiencies, habits and even emotional issues, such as a need for comfort in stressful times.

Take Wendy, for example. A few years ago she came to see me with a full-blown sugar addiction. Her downfall was sugary penny-sweets such as cola bottles and white mice, which she'd buy in little paper bags from her corner shop. It was all rather quaint and seemingly harmless, until she realized that she was going to her local shop so often that it was getting embarrassing! She started to drive around and vary the shops from which she bought her sweets, as she started to feel ashamed of her habit. However, her desire to have them was greater than her shame; she needed her regular sugar fix. She ate them in secret, and she was mortified at the prospect that someone she knew would discover how out of control she was. She was a psychologist, so she was aware that her 'habit' was becoming dangerously addictive. This caused her enormous stress, as she didn't want this part of her private life becoming public.

The truth is that we all have a private and public persona. Have you ever eaten a cream cake at home alone? You wolf it down! However, if you've eaten a cake at the Ritz or another posh hotel, etiquette kicks in and you slow down dramatically – and probably use a delicate little fork as well! I'm a great believer in the idea that a little of what you fancy does you good, but there's a huge difference between being obsessed with particular foods and simply enjoying the pleasure of eating them as a part of a healthy lifestyle.

Wendy is a prime example of what happens when cravings *turn bad*. She overcame her problem by first acknowledging her danger time (i.e., when she was most likely to hit the shops for sweets); we worked out that it was when she was at home studying for her PhD. She wanted something to nibble on and help with the stress – and possibly even to reward her on an unconscious level. So once we had highlighted the danger time, we put steps in place to ensure that she had healthy nibbles to hand – things that were crunchy and satisfying. She made a tomato salsa and ate it with carrots, celery and cucumber, and it's now become her staple 'treat' when she's working. Anything is possible!

What's Your Barcode?

Have you found that no matter *how* hard you work at losing weight, however strict you are with yourself, it is a constant daily struggle with little return? Have you got friends who seem to drop weight with very little effort – or even stay slim and trim on a diet that would make you balloon? There is no doubt that the frustration these scenarios bring can undermine even the most disciplined dieter, and lead many to give up the fight because it just seems hopeless.

You will be interested to learn that there may be good reasons why you are getting stuck. A new type of scientific research, known as epigenetics, suggests that your current likes, dislikes, cravings and even your propensity to put on or ability to lose weight could be down to your mother, father or even your grandmother. Epigenetics is the study of inheritable changes that impact on your genes, without altering your DNA sequence. It transpires that what your ancestors ate in previous generations can affect you now!

Your 'epigenetic' state is like your own unique barcode. Although you may eat exactly the same things as someone else, both bodies will respond differently and part of that is down to generational history. The information generated by this new branch of science is proving to be invaluable in enhancing our understanding of obesity – and our inherited behaviour towards food. So how does this affect you?

> ### Fat mice
>
> According to an article in the *New Scientist,* obese male mice are more likely to father unhealthy off-spring. Their diets cause tiny changes in the 'cellular modification' of their sperm, which may cause metabolic disorders in the baby mice. This discovery brings us closer to understanding how lifestyle choices affect the health of future generations. Your struggle to lose weight might in fact be your parents' fault!

Nature vs Nurture

Do you believe that you were born as a 'blank slate' or do you think you had an in-built predisposition towards the things you have come to like or dislike? How does your relationship with food mirror or differ from that of your parents or your siblings? If it's similar, do you think it has anything to do with what you ate as children or how food was presented or used (for example, was food used for comfort or offered as a treat)? Or do you think that there is something deeper afoot here?

There are two main schools of thought. *Tabula rasa* is a Latin phrase meaning 'blank slate', and it is the name of a branch of science that believes that a child is born 'blank', wholly shaped by his environment. The theory is that an individual becomes who they are through exposure to their environment and their experience of the world.

The other side of the debate is that genetics play a large part in our development, and that we are born with a predisposition to certain behaviours, personalities and intelligence levels as well as inheriting physical traits, such as eye, hair and skin colour. A large part of who we become is, effectively, 'in our genes'.

Genes are our blueprint for life, helping to form our bodies from the moment of conception. They are the 'masters' of creation, and tell our cells how to operate – whether they should become bone or muscle or nerve, for example. Genes are created from protein, and they are switched on or off – or activated or deactivated – to perform their role. Let's say there is a genetic illness in your family. What this means is that the genes that would normally be 'switched on' to protect you will remain 'switched off', making you more at risk of acquiring the disease.

What the study of epigenetics has discovered is that it's not just illnesses and disease that can be passed through generations. Scientists have found that what your mother, father and grandparents ate in the generations prior to your birth can affect which genes are switched on and which genes are not. If you had overweight parents or grandparents, it may well be that your 'fat' gene is switched on, and you will be predisposed to become overweight even if you do not overeat or partake in a lifestyle that will encourage weight gain. We now know, too, that diet, smoking and alcohol intake can cause chemical modifications in the genes that adversely affect their activity and their protein production.

What Does This Mean for You?

The food we eat is broken down into molecules that the body can use. One of the most studied epigenetic processes is DNA methylation. It has been found that a diet high in 'methyl-donating nutrients', which produce the tags that switch certain genes on and off, can positively affect genes. Methyl-donating nutrients include folic acid and the B-complex vitamins. Interestingly, too, the supplement SAM-e

(S-adenosyl methionine) is methyl-donating, and this is significant because this supplement is the synthetic form of a compound created naturally in the body from the amino acid methionine and adenosine triphosphate (ATP) – the energy-producing compound that we discussed earlier (see page 45). It may follow that our ability to produce energy at cell level may be affected by what our ancestors ate! These three elements, B vitamins, folic acid and SAM-e can positively alter our genes when we are in the womb.

This may all sound quite technical, but the upshot is this: if you inherit genes that predispose you to certain diseases or even towards becoming overweight, and you then go on to eat a diet lacking in methyl-donating foods throughout your lifetime, you will be at a greater risk of acquiring these conditions than others.

Epigenetics and the Drop Zone Diet

Epigenetics suggest that the reason why you crave certain foods and reach for specific food types to comfort you when you are vulnerable and stressed could be down to your genes. But does this mean that your destiny is already determined? That your predisposition to excess weight gain is set in stone? The answer is a resounding 'no'. If you make sustained, significant changes to your diet that positively impact upon your genetic make-up, you could affect the health of generations to come. And it's not too late for you, either. Eating a diet rich in methyl-donating foods will help to ensure that faulty gene activation doesn't have such an impact. In other words, just because you have a predisposition towards fat or eating fatty foods for comfort, doesn't mean that you *have* to be that way. Eating methyl-donating foods can affect the way our genes operate *now*, and make us less susceptible to genetic influences. The very good news is that the foods on the Drop Zone Diet are high in methyl-donating nutrients, helping to overcome problems that you may have inherited.

Generations to come

> Choosing a healthy diet and lifestyle won't only impact upon your health and wellbeing now, but will also affect your children and their children. According to Dr Catherine Suter from the Victor Chang Cardiac Research Institute, 'We don't need long-term generational genetic changes. It only takes one generation of dietary change to revert the genes back to healthy genes.' You could be making life a lot easier for generations to come by taking control of your own health now.

When Things Become Unbalanced

My mother used to say, 'A place for everything and everything in its place', and I like to think our bodies operate in the same way. Each and every bit of us has form and function, and is connected to and dependent upon all of our other 'bits' to achieve survival. There is *synergy* in our bodies. Our organs and cells react and respond to minute changes both internally and externally; as a species our survival and evolution is totally reliant upon this delicate interplay.

Our bodies strive to maintain 'homeostasis' (stable, constant conditions, or a state of balance) by regulating the internal environment. Examples of the mechanisms that are designed to do this include regulation of temperature and pH, and the constant flow of the circulatory system. One of the main influences on the smooth functioning of every single operation in the body is the food we eat.

If you eat junk, your internal self-regulating systems will aim to get rid of the by-products and toxins through numerous routes of elimination. For example, if you eat too much salt, much of the excess will be excreted via the kidneys through your urine. But what happens if you take in more toxins than your body can effectively expel at any one time? Does this cause a 'back-up'? Does it 'clog us up'? Does our body become less efficient because it is too busy trying to keep up with all the elimination that needs to happen?

Well, sort of . . . While our bodies can still capably do their jobs, there is extra pressure placed on all of our organs. Our bodies effectively have to work that much harder just to maintain the equilibrium. It's not rocket science to understand that if an organ is overworked, it becomes tired and less efficient. Even when you are just sitting and watching TV – and your body is relatively still – underneath your skin your 'working mechanisms' are going like the clappers in an attempt to keep your physiology on its correct axis and to maintain homeostasis. When it's clogged with junk, even the strongest body will struggle, and you may experience this through symptoms such as fatigue, stress, coughs and colds, headaches, an irritable bowel, low sex drive and, of course, lack of energy.

The World Health Organization has classified these non-specific symptoms as 'adrenal exhaustion'. Adrenal exhaustion is, therefore, characterized by a series of seemingly random symptoms that make you feel exhausted and ill to the point that you secretly worry that there's something seriously wrong with you. In fact, your body is depleted and fatigued. When you are exhausted in this way, you are much more likely to crave certain foods in an attempt to shift your energy and mood. In reality, however, the foods you're craving aren't usually what's required. What you really need – what you are really searching for – is a 'pick-me-up'.

Mood and energy levels *definitely* impact upon your food choices and even your relationship to food. Let's try to work out why you crave a particular food.

Understanding Food Cravings

Answer the following questions to establish your unique relationship with cravings and specific foods. If more than one answer seems appropriate, choose the one that seems to apply most often.

Section one: the comfort food snacker

You crave fatty foods and warming comfort foods like takeaways. Do you:

a) Think about food most of the time?
b) Feel tired most of the time, including when waking in the morning?
c) Have low energy levels?
d) Have problems focusing and concentrating on one task?
e) Feel too exhausted to go to the gym and work out?
f) Feel mentally depleted (i.e. head-stressed, with too much to think about)?
g) Feel frustrated because you are constantly exhausted and run down?

Section two: the savoury food snacker

You crave salty, savoury snacks such as crisps, nuts and cheese. Do you:

a) Have a battle in your head every night *not* to pig out?
b) Experience erratic mood swings when you are pre-menstrual?
c) Find it difficult to switch off and relax, even in bed?
d) Obsess about food (when/what you will eat next time)?
e) Eat unconsciously (suddenly the whole packet is gone)?
f) Have intermittent periods of depression or anxiety?
g) Eat in spurts (binge then fast, binge then fast)?

Section three: the stress-head food snacker

You crave sweets, chocolate, caffeine and alcohol. Do you:

a) Have an addictive personality (want more and more and more)?
b) Do 20 things at once and are always on the go?
c) Rely on coffee, cola and alcohol to get through the day/evening?
d) Smoke cigarettes or cannabis?
e) Forget things, like what you ate for dinner last night?
f) Find that you have gone off sex?
g) Find your mind wandering off when people are talking to you?

Section four: the emotional food snacker

You sometimes feel ashamed or guilty after eating. Do you:

a) Hide food or lie about what you've eaten?
b) Eat until you feel nauseous?

c) Eat alone or in secret?

d) Eat to release emotions?

e) Find that your relationship with food interferes with your life?

f) Soothe painful emotions through food?

g) Get more pleasure from food than anything else?

Section one

If you answered 'yes' to most of the questions in this section, I suspect you tend to turn to food to get some instant energy in your life. Consider the following:

Dilemma	Solution	Cravings	Positive health action*
You are trapped in a cycle of energy and fatigue, experiencing almost chronic fatigue and low energy levels. This impacts upon your motivation to the point where you just can't be bothered even trying to make positive change any more. In fact, you've probably asked yourself many times over, 'What's the point?' Why try once again when you've made half-hearted attempts in the past and each time you have failed?	The Drop Zone Diet will help you to get out of this vicious cycle once and for all, giving you quick results in a short space of time. You need this to kick-start your motivation. Once you've got the passion and energy back in your life you can set yourself short-term goals, such as joining a gym or going walking with friends, so you don't become overwhelmed by apathy again.	Your craving for fatty foods is actually a desire to get some energy into your body. Fat contains more calories than protein or carbs and therefore feeds your low energy and also acts as a comforter. You need to choose foods high in natural healthy fats such as salmon, mackerel, nuts and avocados. See the list below (pages 61–2) for more information on curbing fatty foods cravings.	Swimming
			Horse riding
			Cycling
			Massage

* Your positive health action will involve exercise where you are supported and upheld by 'something', such as water, a bicycle or a horse. You don't have much energy and are constantly exhausted, so allowing something else to take the majority of the strain will provide you with support, while allowing you to move. Deep-tissue or lymphatic-drainage massage will enhance your 'recovery' tremendously by encouraging relaxation and the removal of toxins that may be causing you to feel sluggish.

Section two

If you answered 'yes' to most of the questions in this section, then it's likely that you have quite an addictive relationship with food. You love it and loathe it in equal measure at times. Consider the following:

Dilemma	Solution	Cravings	Positive health action*
You are a bit of a control freak and a perfectionist and the fact that you cannot gain control over your eating habits causes you stress with a capital 'S'. Your desire for perfection and the 'perfect body' is currently out of your control as your cravings dictate the state of your health and size of your body. As salt absorbs water you probably suffer from water retention, making you feel bloated and sluggish.	There is a well-known saying that 'Where salt goes, water will follow'. Water neutralizes the acidic effect of eating too much salt, which ultimately culminates in high blood pressure and disease. The Drop Zone Diet is high in alkalizing foods – foods that help to create balance as they naturally contain the correct sodium/water ratio that your body requires. Releasing excess fluids/fats will speed up your weight loss so that you get quick and easy results.	If you are eating high-salt foods, you are likely to be eating a lot of highly processed foods and snacks. There is not even one food, in its natural form, that contains too much salt. Electrolyte-containing foods, such as carrots, broccoli, kale and cabbage will provide the vital salts and minerals required for a healthy body and help in the removal of toxins. See the list below (pages 61–2) for more information on curbing salt cravings.	Golf
			Squash
			Chess
			Photography

* Fun, competitive exercise where you endeavour to perfect your technique against a partner will benefit you. Chilled-out exercise would be too boring for you and you would simply give up after a while. You need exercise that is mentally stimulating and challenging, in order to engage your brain. Photography would also work well to bring out your creativity and satisfy your artistic nature.

Section three

If you answered 'yes' to most of the questions in this section, then you probably have a stressful lifestyle and use food/drink as an 'upper and downer'. Consider the following:

Dilemma	Solution	Cravings	Positive health action*
Your endocrine (hormone) system is out of kilter. The endocrine system influences every single cell in the body and is highly involved in mood regulation and metabolism. The adrenal glands are part of the endocrine system and your adrenal glands could be exhausted and depleted due to stress and a busy lifestyle. These glands release cortisol in response to stress, a hormone required for use in an emergency. They are supposed to switch on and off according to the severity of impending danger (i.e., a sabre-toothed tiger). Your adrenal glands are switched on almost permanently due to worry and stress. This leaves them depleted and you exhausted.	Feeding the body to replenish and nurture the endocrine system will have an enormous impact on your health and energy levels. Your body needs to be soothed – bathed in nutrients that will restock your energy supplies. Get your energy larder jam-packed again so that when you do genuinely need an extra boost of energy to get you through the day, you have it in spades within your body rather than having to kick-start it with a sugar snack. The structure of the sugar molecule (sucrose + fructose) places a burden not only on the pancreas but also the liver too. Removing excess sugar from your diet will stop the crash-bang energy highs and lows you currently experience.	Complex carbohydrates will support your transition from exhaustion to energy. Taking the pressure off your pancreas is critical to reduce your propensity towards diabetes. Including whole brown rice as a staple in your diet three times a week will improve your health significantly. Brown rice helps the brain to manufacture 'GABA' – a neurotransmitter that 'mops up' cortisol from your bloodstream and supports its speedy elimination from your body, leaving you feeling peaceful and relaxed.	Yoga / Meditation / T'ai chi / Walking

* Create balance through activities that support your body (i.e., low-impact exercise and stretching) rather than high-impact, adrenaline-producing exercises that will deplete you even further. Meditative exercises such as t'ai chi and yoga can help to calm the mind, centre the body and lead you back to harmony, building up endurance and flexibility in stages, to make you strong from the inside out.

Section four

If you answered 'yes' to most of the questions in this section, then food may have become a disproportionate source of comfort for you during emotional or challenging times. Consider the following:

Dilemma	Solution	Cravings	Positive health action*
You have a strong psychological association with food and have probably used it as a friend, a crutch and a comforter throughout difficult periods in your life. This form of emotional eating can impact on self-esteem as the bigger you get, the more away from 'you' you become. In order to suppress these negative emotions, as well as the guilt and shame you feel about eating junk, you eat more comfort foods, which ultimately creates a vicious circle. People in this group are often highly intelligent and struggle with the dichotomy between knowing how to live their ideal life, and the life they are currently living. This causes more pain and discomfort, which perpetuates the cycle.	The spiritual teacher Gary Zukav says, 'True authentic empowerment is when your personality is in alignment with your soul.' How beautiful a truth that is. Emotional eating can occur when, somewhere along the line, we lose our authentic 'self', and feel bereft, alone and frightened. The soups on the Drop Zone Diet will provide nourishment for you as they feed your senses as well as your body. I call them soups for the soul because they fulfil the body's core need for rich, nurturing foods that are easy to digest and also strengthen the central nervous system to soothe and balance the body.	If the outer casing of your body, your flesh, isn't a true reflection of the inner you, you will always be at odds with yourself. Foods to soothe and heal the body for you would include yellow, orange, red and purple foods that are rich in antioxidants that will help to purify your body. They will also make you feel full of colour, turning up your natural vibration and increasing your energy to a new level. It's almost like your body takes on the hue of these foods and you go from a sense of darkness into the light.	Writing/poetry
			Choir/singing
			Musical instruments
			Dance

* An expressive outlet would be perfect for you and one such as writing is ideal. Why not Google writing clubs in your area, or look for poetry classes so that you can begin to get your emotions on paper? Beautiful sounds and movement would also be great, so joining a choir, playing that musical instrument you've always promised yourself you'd learn, or joining a dance class at your local gym would work wonders for you.

Satisfying the Itch

Cravings make us impulsive and cause us to behave irrationally. Gone is the professional, chic career woman or the doting, caring father. It's now every man for himself, as the need to satisfy the 'itch' overwhelms rhyme, reason and logic. To help you through those dark hours, I've put together a list of the top 10 cravings I have seen in my clinic over the past decade, and offer healthy alternative solutions. If you get a craving that is driving you crazy, try to satisfy it from a nutritional point of view rather than reverting to your old habits. This list is worth carrying with you at all times. While you are on the Drop Zone Diet, you'll need to be careful not to add too many extras to the plan. It's an extreme diet that works most effectively when you stick to it religiously. But the chances are that you simply won't experience your usual cravings because the diet is so well balanced, and your increased energy levels will give you the get-up-and-go you need to show those cravings straight out of the door.

	Craving	Your body may really want	Healthier option
1	Chocolate	Magnesium, B vitamins, theobromine (an element found in cocoa that works like caffeine on the body), dopamine (a neurotransmitter that controls the 'reward and pleasure' part of the brain)	• Handful of mixed nuts with cranberries • Steamed spinach with fresh lemon juice • Handful of cherries
2	Sweets	Chromium (see page 122), phosphorous (essential for the production of ATP (see page 45)), and serotonin (the feel-good neurotransmitter)	• Hot water and lemon juice with 1 teaspoon of honey • Fresh homemade natural popcorn • 3 rice cakes with a (very) light spreading of Nutella hazelnut spread

	Craving	Your body may really want	Healthier option
3	Fizzy drinks	Calcium, glucose, epinephrine (adrenaline)	• Coconut water • Diluted fresh juice in sparkling mineral water
4	Coffee	Iron, dopamine, epinephrine (adrenaline)	• Single decaf espresso, black • Small skimmed milk decaf latte • Handful of pecan nuts • Small tomato juice with a dash of Worcestershire sauce
5	Bread	Carbohydrates, calcium, iron	• Ryvita crispbread • 1 grated carrot with fresh lemon juice and raisins • 5 steamed asparagus spears with fresh lime juice
6	Alcohol	Glucose, magnesium, zinc	• 1 small boiled egg • Handful of pumpkin seeds in 2 tablespoons of natural yoghurt • Sparking water with fresh lime juice
7	Cheese	Calcium, sodium, protein	• 1 beef tomato sliced and grilled, eaten on 2 rice cakes • 1 carrot or 2 celery sticks, chopped • 50g cottage cheese with the above
8	Crisps	Iodine, sodium, serotonin	• Roasted cabbage (chopped seaweed style) • Fresh carrot, apple and ginger juice • 3 rice cakes with a (very) thin spreading of hummus
9	Pasta	Carbohydrates, potassium, magnesium	• A small banana • 100g toasted tofu • 2 rice cakes with 50g cottage cheese
10	Evening munchies	Chromium, serotonin, fats	• Fresh homemade natural popcorn • Crudités • 3 rice cakes with a (very) light spreading of hummus or Nutella hazelnut spread

Life-saving craving

> Does your body really crave foods that contain nutrients that it lacks? What is the basis for these cravings and where does habit meet science and biochemistry? For Elsie Campbell, responding to her unique craving probably saved her life. Elsie developed an uncontrollable craving for iceberg lettuce, to the point where she would come home from work and head straight to the fridge and eat a whole lettuce in one sitting. Thankfully, Elsie's husband is a scientist and he recognized that these cravings might have something to do with compounds in the lettuce – in this case, sulforaphane, a chemical that attacks cancer cells. Sure enough, Elsie went to her GP and was diagnosed with breast cancer. This early detection meant that Elsie's cancer was successfully treated. In this case, a craving was no bad thing!

Listen to your body when you experience cravings, and try to give it a healthy dose of exactly what it really needs. It is possible to be dedicated and determined to meet your weight-loss goals and still enjoy foods that will support your emotional health and physical requirements. The Drop Zone Diet will help you to develop a taste for healthy alternatives to your current unhealthy choices, and its careful biochemical construction means that your body soon won't be crying out for treats as it did in the past.

Most dieters worry that an extreme diet will cause blood-sugar drops and they'll lose the will to continue when the uncontrollable urges, bad moods and shakiness sets in. Rest assured, the Drop Zone Diet is going to *smooth* you out so that you feel steady, calm and full of vital energy. Let's find out how.

CHAPTER 4

The One Where We Get You on an Even Keel

Do you become a different person when you need sugar? Do you become ratty, irritable and moody – perhaps even shaky? Are you worried about starting new a diet because you are afraid that you'll become a monster for its duration, alienating your family and friends and feeling completely miserable? This may have been your experience in the past, but I can assure you that the Drop Zone Diet is completely different. Your energy levels will be constant throughout the day – every day – instead of peaking and troughing like the graphs on an ECG machine.

The battle to eat healthily and stick to your diet versus the *need* to eat sugar is a fierce one. The chances are that you've experienced cravings that were so strong you've been knocked completely off kilter. Is sugar *really* so additive, or is this more about our need to occupy ourselves with constant distractions – food being one of them?

'If I don't eat sugar or chocolate every day, I get the shakes. I crave it and have a mental battle with myself until I eventually give in and go to the vending machine at work for a fix. Then I hate myself for being weak. I'm desperate to lose weight, but when the craving is so strong, I'm so overwhelmed that it consumes me.'

A True Addiction

According to Dr John Hoebel and his colleagues at Princeton University in America, sugar is as addictive as heroin. Hoebel and his team discovered that rats who normally had a diet that was made up of about 25 per cent sugar experienced shaking, chattering teeth and signs of anxiety when sugar was removed from their diet. When the rats were forced to go cold turkey, their symptoms were synonymous with those of people who were experiencing heroin withdrawal.

Could you be addicted to sugar? Answer the following questions:

1. I get the shakes if I don't eat for three hours (or less)
2. I have significant energy dips throughout the day
3. I become clumsy and drop or bang into things
4. I become forgetful and sometimes can't remember what I had for dinner the previous day
5. I feel faint and light-headed at times, especially when standing up
6. I always crave 'something sweet' after dinner
7. I get irritable when I haven't had my sugar fix
8. I need sugar to give me an energy boost mid-afternoon
9. I have a sweet stash in the car, at work and at home, and panic if I don't have some at hand – just in case
10. Once I start eating biscuits, I can't just have one or two – I have to eat the whole packet

If you answered yes to three or more of the above scenarios, then it's highly likely that you have an addiction to sugar.

Later in this book (see page 207) I'll tell you how to reduce the amount of sugar you take in – with no sense that you are 'doing without' and no withdrawal symptoms – for the duration of your diet. However, it is worth noting here that if you are a sugar addict and have a history of diabetes in your family, you will need to consider very seriously how you are going to replace sugars in your diet in the long-term, and you should consult with your doctor to avoid going down the same route as other family members.

You may be wondering at this point why sugar is so bad, and why an addiction to something so innocuous should be cause for concern. There are serious grounds for worry – not just to do with weight, which is severely impacted, but also to do with overall health, wellbeing and even appearance.

Dr Kathleen DesMaisons is author of the book *Potatoes not Prozac*, and she claims that if sugar had been discovered for the first time today, it would be unlikely to get past the health authorities. She first became aware of issues surrounding sugar when she was running a drug and alcohol addiction clinic. She recognized that the alcoholics she was treating were also sugar addicts. By adding a series of key nutrients and removing the sugar from their diets (as well as supporting this removal within their treatment programme), she was successful in treating 92 per cent of the alcoholics – even those who were 'hard core'.

We now know that sugar is both physically and mentally addictive, and there is plenty of evidence to suggest that it can be harmful to health in large quantities. In 2011, childhood obesity expert Robert Lustig claimed that sugar contributes to 35 million deaths a year worldwide. He called for it to be taxed in a similar way to alcohol and cigarettes due to its toxic impact on health. He argues that sugar not only makes people fat, but it also raises blood pressure, affects hormone production (and hormonal balance) and is implicated in many life-threatening diseases such as diabetes and heart disease. Your chocolate biscuit addiction may be more dangerous than you thought. So what exactly does sugar do?

Tooth decay and heart disease

We all know that sugar rots our teeth, but did you know that a result of tooth decay and poor gum health is heart disease? Bleeding gums allow bacteria to gain entry to your bloodstream and stick to the platelets in your blood, which can cause clots. Clots block arteries and prevent blood flow to and from the heart – which can lead to a heart attack.

Suppressed immunity

The immune system is weakened by excessive sugar consumption. It's interesting to note that vitamin C and sugar have very similar chemical structures. Vitamin C is required to support the immune system (as well as other systems in the body); however, when too much sugar enters the bloodstream vitamin C has to battle with sugar to enter the cells and more sugar than vitamin C gets in. That impacts upon our ability to fight off disease. And there's more: sugar raises insulin levels, which inhibits the release of growth hormones. In turn, this depresses the immune system. Poor wound healing and cellular repair result from this.

Blood-sugar problems

Diabetes is fast becoming the disease of the century, with around 285 million people currently living with Type 2 diabetes worldwide. In Type 2 diabetes, the pancreas may produce insulin, but the body becomes resistant to it. When you eat foods containing sugars and your blood-glucose levels rise, your pancreas releases insulin to help lower the glucose levels; if your body has become resistant to insulin, your blood-sugar levels stay too high for too long. Diabetes is a chronic disease and every week in the UK about 100 people have a foot amputated because of it. It's also the biggest cause of blindness in the country.

Poor memory

How is your short-term memory? Diets high in refined sugar affect an area of the brain called the hippocampus, which is responsible for memory function. In studies, animals fed on a diet high in refined sugar for between two and 24 months showed decreased levels in the important proteins responsible for brain plasticity and memory formation. Sugar also inhibits the expression of BDNF (Brain-derived neurotrophic factor), which is crucial for the development of new brain tissue and neural pathways. Low levels of BDNF affect the functionality and formation of new brain cells, causing shrinkage and atrophy. And the damage can take place in as little as two months!

Bring on old age

Who wants to look old before their time? Aren't most of us spending a fortune trying to look younger? Well, sugar makes you age more quickly. If health warnings don't scare you off, maybe vanity will! Researchers from Leiden University Medical Centre in association with Unilever UK demonstrated a link between high blood sugar and facial ageing, proving that a high sugar diet makes you look older. A group of individual assessors were shown pictures of men and women with varying blood-sugar levels. The results showed that for every mm/l increase in blood sugar the person was perceived to be five months older!

One Lump or Two (On Your Hips, That Is . . .)?

When you eat sugar it triggers fat storage in the body, and the hormone insulin is released. *Any* type of sugar, from sweets, chocolate, fruit and honey to potatoes and rice triggers this release. The greater the quantity of sugar, the greater the amount of insulin released. Insulin helps to regulate blood-sugar levels and acts, in particular, on the cells of your liver, your muscles and on fat cells, triggering them to absorb glucose, fatty acids and amino acids (the building blocks of protein) from the food you've just eaten. Your body converts the sugar into glucose and glycogen, to be stored in the liver for later use; however, if you raise your blood-sugar levels too high in one sitting, insulin instructs your body to store any excess sugar as fat. The insulin takes up the excess sugars and places them into fat cells, which then become nicely plump.

How your body then stores this fat – whether on the hips or round the abdomen – depends on your particular shape, and this is partly down to genetics, according to Cecilia Lindgren of the Wellcome Trust Centre for Human Genetics at Oxford University. Other factors that affect the amount of fat stored in specific areas include hormones (in particular, oestrogen), age, smoking, alcohol intake, diet and stress (yes, stress makes you fat; see page 109). And it does matter *where* fat is stored. Fat stored around the abdomen is much more dangerous (and linked to far more diseases) than fat stored around the hips. Either way, excess fat is not a good thing, no matter how you look at it.

Fat is not just unattractive; it is alive and awash with cells that create damaging chemicals that have been implicated in a host of serious diseases. For example, scientists have found that subcutaneous fat, which develops around the waist, contains hormones that are biologically active. It releases chemicals called cytokines that make the body more resistant to insulin and also cause low-level inflammation throughout the body that can increase the risk of heart disease. Your tummy overhang could also make you more prone to diabetes.

If you don't want to become a statistic, then you need to take control of your diet and make lasting health changes. Unfortunately women are more prone to excess abdominal subcutaneous fat, especially as they go through the menopause. Their ratio of fat to lean tissue shifts and for some women, despite sticking to a healthy diet, fat will accumulate around their mid-section. If your waist is bigger than 35 inches (89cm), you have an increased risk of health problems. In men, a waist bigger than 40 inches (102cm) indicates the same.

Red alert!

You have over 10,000 taste buds in your mouth! Sweetness is detected by protein receptors within the taste buds found at the front and back of your tongue. Interesting, the colour of a food *can* affect its sweetness. Red foods have up to 10 per cent more impact on your receptors than other foods! If you are craving something sweet, go red! Cherry tomatoes are a fabulous on-the-go snack and they'll feed your senses, too.

Thankfully, the body does tend to utilize abdominal fat for energy before it breaks down fat from other areas, such as the hips and thighs. Cutting down on sugar and eating a diet that is rich in complex rather than simple carbohydrates can help to reduce the amount of stored fat anywhere in the body, and that's one reason why the Drop Zone Diet is so successful. Not only is it packed with foods designed to reduce inflammation and support balanced blood-sugar levels, but it takes the pressure off *all* of your organs, thus lowering the risks associated with subcutaneous fat.

Changing Your Palate

As part of your evolution from sugar addict to stress-free, healthy, slim beauty, you will need to redefine your palate. Many of us have become so used to foods with very high levels of sugar, salt and fat that natural, simple, whole foods can seem bland and dull in comparison. The truth is that lovely, unrefined and unprocessed foods offer a delicious range of subtle textures, flavours and tastes that will get your senses tingling! You just need to reawaken your senses in order to appreciate them once again. The beauty of developing a refined palate is that healthy foods suddenly take on a life of their own – and their vibrancy imbues you with life as well! They become a delight to eat instead of a chore and you'll find yourself gravitating towards them instead of your usual sweet treats as soon as your palate is restored.

During the first few days of the Drop Zone Diet you may find yourself bewildered by these fresh, new tastes. The biochemical construction of the diet means that you won't actually crave the unhealthy foods you used to eat, but it may take a little time for your taste buds to spring back into action and recognize the wonderful, yet more subtle, flavours with which you are presenting them. The Drop Zone Diet does contain sugars, but it depends upon natural sugars such as honey, fruit and even some vegetables to provide you with energy. Rather than go 'cold turkey' by removing all sugar from your diet, you'll be offered gentle, natural sweetness to keep the hunger pangs at bay and make cravings a thing of the past. The combination of a host of fresh, nutrient-dense foods and a low calorie intake means you'll lose more weight, more quickly than you ever thought possible. Better still, your palate will slowly adjust to appreciate healthy foods so that when you finish your 14-day stint, you'll be ready for more!

There is one sugar we haven't discussed in detail, and removing it from your diet is paramount to the Drop Zone Diet's success. Have you guessed what that is? Yes, it's alcohol and yes, you *can* do without it. Here's why.

CHAPTER 5

The One Where
We Cut Out the Booze!

How random is your knowledge of diets and health? Where do the diets you have done in the past come from, and how did you find out about them? I suspect that very often friends, colleagues and family have raved about the latest diets on the market, and those are the ones you chose. That's fine. But ask yourself this: Are the people who supply you with this information always on a diet? By definition, are they failing to achieve long-term success? To achieve *sustainable* long-term success, you need to turn your attention – and listen – to people who have mastered it already.

Successful people leave clues! All you need to do is find someone you admire on the health and wellness front and then model their behaviour. My own role model, in terms of looking healthy, vibrant and beautiful, is Jennifer Aniston. I believe I can state quite categorically that Jennifer Aniston 'does not eat all the pies'! Instead she has a dedicated fitness regime and eats a healthy, well-balanced diet. I also suspect that she likes to have fun, kick back once in a while, perhaps eat a Mexican meal and have the odd tequila! A little bit of what you fancy does you good and I'm a great believer in laughter being the best medicine. A fantastic night out with your friends, lots of giggles and laughter, great food and a little wine complement a healthy, balanced lifestyle.

Yes, wine is fine from time to time, and alcohol can have

a host of benefits when drunk in moderation, and in combination with a good diet. However, for a small period of time you are going to need to abstain. Giving up alcohol is a critical part of the Drop Zone Diet and it is essential to its success. I'm under no illusions about the problems that many people have with giving up, and I realize that this is the part of the diet that may cause you to struggle the most. No alcohol for 14 days! What will you do without booze at the weekend? How will you unwind at the end of the day?

The truth is that alcohol has become such an intrinsic part of our lives that envisaging a 'dry' period, regardless of its duration, can fill people with dread. However, I also know that by purchasing this book you are searching for better health and a balanced weight; I know that you are looking for a lifestyle that is compatible with the way you want to *live*. The Drop Zone Diet will be an integral part of your evolution from feeling overweight and tired all the time to becoming svelte, energized and looking and feeling great.

So Why Drop Alcohol?

Drinking alcohol slows down the metabolism of body fats. Your body transforms alcohol into acetate – a unit of energy that it then uses as your body's primary source of fuel, instead of burning your fat for energy. In other words, when you drink, the alcohol is metabolized while the energy from the other food you eat is laid down as fat. You will store fat more quickly, even if you aren't even eating that much. The *American Journal of Clinical Nutrition* recently demonstrated that fat metabolism is reduced by as much as 73 per cent after only two drinks of vodka and lemonade over a one-hour period (that's equivalent to two small glasses of wine), effectively shutting down the body's ability to access fat stores. These are the very fats that we are intending to break down and get out of your system over the course of the diet, so if you drink alcohol you are putting a large spanner in the works and slowing down the whole fat-removal process. A few drinks can mean that your fat loss is stalled for hours; excessive drinking can stall the process for days.

Where Did the Fat Come From?

Your body will never work against you; it always does the best it can with what you give it. So the excess fat you are carrying is basically an energy store from which you can derive energy at any point that you may need it. It's a bank of fuel stacked in the cells of subcutaneous fat (the fat that you can grab hold of – in other words, the inch you can pinch around your waist). Somewhere along the line you have eaten more calories than your body needed to burn at that moment in time and your body converted those excess calories from sugar into fat throughout a complex chemical process called fatty acid synthesis.

Fatty acid synthesis (FAS) occurs when your blood-glucose levels are high – after eating a high-carbohydrate meal, for example – and the hormone insulin gets involved in the whole process. Most people know that insulin, manufactured by the pancreas, is involved in the regulation of blood sugars but what you may not know is that it also plays a significant role in metabolism of fats and fuels to store for future use (subcutaneous fat) or use for energy (fuel) now. Insulin initiates an enzyme called fatty acid synthase, which regulates the rate at which your body stores fat.

To ensure you get the most out of the Drop Zone Diet we

have to take the pressure off the pancreas (and its job of manufacturing insulin) by giving your body a reduced calorie intake *and* taking out alcohol altogether. In this way, the fat that is already stored is fully accessible for quick and easy breakdown.

So, armed with the information that removing alcohol from your diet will help you lose weight more quickly, how easy will it be for you to eliminate alcohol from your life for 14 days? Does the thought bring you out in a cold sweat?

The husband

My wife is always on and off diets like a yo-yo and, in all honesty, I switched off listening to her go on about how fat she was years ago. I just don't see it. I love her and to me she is beautiful. But last year an illness meant that she was on medication that did contribute to gaining excess weight over a short period of time. I too had reached the big 'four-oh' and felt heavy around my middle. She suggested that we do the Drop Zone Diet together and support each other to achieve a much healthier lifestyle. I really thought I'd miss the alcohol, but I can honestly say that I didn't. Although I don't drink much anyway, when something's taken from you it can make you want it even more. However, from Day 1 the Drop Zone Diet was a breeze (admittedly my wife made all the soups) and we had a good laugh making the smoothies and juices. I didn't even notice the missing booze. I lost 17 pounds (my wife lost 13) and we were both staggered by how easy it was. I have started exercising more regularly and have kept the weight off. I'm chuffed to bits!

A Nation of Addicts?

According to the NHS statistics and data analytics information centre, there were 160,181 prescriptions written for drugs to help treat addiction to alcohol in 2010. Studies have found that alcohol misuse is rapidly increasing (particularly among young women), and it has become a problem for many of us.

Perhaps it's the way we look at it. In her book, *Why French Women Don't Get Fat*, Mireille Guiliano points out that the French view wine as liquid food, with calories, nutrients and flavours. French children are raised to respect alcohol and to view it as something to be enjoyed, not abused. Adults in France don't binge on alcohol as it 'dulls the senses' and invariably dulls the taste and enjoyment of food. They know what we should know: too much alcohol causes us to eat more and it can take a lot longer for us to feel satisfied. Hence the problem with overeating and excess weight!

Drunkorexia

Conflicting pressures to stay slim but still partake in an ever-expanding drinking culture has lead to the term 'drunkorexia', which is particularly prevalent among young women in the UK. The craze of limiting food intake in order to make more room for alcohol consumption is particularly virulent amongst university students and young women between the ages of 18 and 20, who often 'store up' their calorie allowance by eating as little as possible (if anything) during the day, in order to drink heavily in the evenings and not gain weight.

This is a seriously dangerous practice. The body requires nutrition to function at optimum level, so on top of dealing with inadequate nutrition, it then has to deal with the toxins (poisons) created by binge drinking. In particular it puts enormous strain on the liver, heart and brain and has many very serious health implications. The irony is that weight gain *will* eventually occur anyway, because the body will go into overdrive and store everything that is eaten as fat, and the alcohol will then prevent it from being released for energy.

So Are You Drinking Too Much?

A dependency on alcohol can creep up on you and catch you unawares. Your patterns of drinking can alter subtly over time and a soothing drink to help unwind after a hard day can become a 'must-have' stress reliever before you know it.

Are you on the cusp of living the life you want to live, but alcohol is dragging you down? Does any of this sound familiar?

- I drink until I go to bed, waking up feeling more tired the next morning and needing sugar
- I am used to waking with a hangover at weekends
- I have a mental battle whether to buy alcohol or not
- I decided never to drink at home but broke that resolution many times
- I made a decision not to drink on school nights but break this all the time
- I frequently go for a drink after work to wind down
- I regularly socialize with my colleagues straight after work

This quiz will help you to establish exactly where you are in relation to alcohol right now:

1. You are home, and it's around dinnertime. You feel tempted to drink but you do not have any alcohol. Do you . . .
   a) Eat dinner and resist going out for a few drinks?
   b) Eat dinner and then perhaps go out later for a few drinks?
   c) Immediately go out to the shops and buy some alcohol to bring back home to drink with dinner?
   d) Immediately go out for a few drinks and get something to eat at a local bar or restaurant?
   e) Skip dinner altogether and go out drinking?

2. You are out shopping, and you notice that your favourite alcoholic beverage is on sale. Assuming you have the money, do you . . .
   a) Notice the sale but feel no desire at all to buy alcohol?
   b) Notice the sale and, although you are tempted, resist the temptation to buy alcohol just because it's on sale?
   c) Buy a small quantity to save a little money?
   d) Buy a medium quantity so you can save a fair amount of money, and also have a supply at home?
   e) Buy a large quantity so you can save a lot of money, and also have a large supply at home?

3. You are out with friends. You've had one small drink, and you're thinking about leaving so you can

drive safely. Your friends want you to stay and continue drinking. Do you . . .

a) Avoid the situation in the first place by not drinking alcohol before driving?

b) Tell them that you've had enough, thanks anyway, and then leave?

c) Stay longer, but only have non-alcoholic drinks?

d) Tell them that you'll stay for just another couple of drinks, but then you need to go?

e) Stay as long as they do, knowing that you can out-drink them and still get home safely?

4. You have a splitting headache after drinking too much last night. Since your body is having withdraw symptoms, do you . . .

a) Not recognize this scenario? You avoid getting a headache in the first place by only having one or two drinks the night before, or not drinking at all.

b) Learn from your mistake, and vow to never again drink to the point that you have a headache the following day?

c) Take the day off from drinking, take some paracetamol and go back to bed?

d) Take paracetamol to help you feel better as soon as possible, because you're likely to be drinking again later tonight?

e) Try to 'bite back what bit you' by drinking alcohol and seeing if the headache goes away?

5. You are constantly tired and decide to go to the doctor to see if something is physically wrong. The

doctor asks you how much you drink during the course of a week. Do you . . .

a) Tell the truth, and vow to change your habits to become healthier and have more energy?

b) Admit to drinking too much, but not to as many drinks as you actually have because you're embarrassed?

c) Admit to drinking too much, but joke about it with the doctor?

d) Tell the doctor that you only have a couple of drinks now and then, even though you drink nearly every day?

e) Admit to drinking a lot, but ignore your doctor's advice to cut back because you don't see it as a problem?

6. Your family or significant other is pressuring you to quit or cut back on drinking alcohol. Do you . . .

a) Take their advice because they are more important than alcohol?

b) Cut back a little bit right away, and plan to cut back more in the future?

c) Try to cut back, but can't because you find it very difficult?

d) Drink as much as you ever did, but try to keep it hidden?

e) Ignore them because you enjoy getting drunk?

7. Your spouse's parents will be staying with you for a couple of weeks. They do not drink and your

spouse wants you to avoid drinking around them.
Do you . . .

a) Completely avoid drinking while they are there
   because alcohol doesn't mean anything to you?
b) Cut back drastically while they are around?
c) Continue to drink, but do so in secret so no one
   notices?
d) Drink in front of them so they learn to be more
   accepting of your habits?
e) Continue to drink as much as ever because it's
   your life, not theirs?

8. Your friend was nearly in a car accident, and was
   picked up for drink driving. Do you . . .
   a) Vow to never drink alcohol before driving?
   b) Change your habits so you don't get caught up in
      the same thing?
   c) Thank God that it wasn't you because you often
      drive while intoxicated?
   d) Be more aware of the police when you drive so
      they don't catch you?
   e) Laugh about it when you see your friend?

9. You haven't drunk alcohol in a week. Your friends
   are having a party and you're invited. You decide to
   go, but do you . . .
   a) Avoid drinking any alcohol because you've noticed
      how much better you feel and look when sober?
   b) Have just a couple of drinks and then stop,
      because you enjoy being in control of your life?
   c) Drink a little more than you should, but resist the
      urge to get totally drunk?

    d) Drink too much and feel guilty afterwards?

    e) Drink as much as you can to make up for the days you missed?

10. Your friends and family confront you, and they are trying to get you into a rehab or detox programme. Do you . . .

    a) Break down and admit that you need help with this problem?

    b) Admit that you need help, but feel scared because you're not sure you can stop drinking?

    c) Admit that you need help, but feel defensive that other people are ganging up on you?

    d) Get angry because other people are trying to control your life?

    e) Refuse to seek any help because you do not have an alcohol addiction?

Scoring

Add up your answers to the questions using the following point system:

    a) 5 points

    b) 4 points

    c) 3 points

    d) 2 points

    e) 1 point

How did you do?

40–50 points: Congratulations! You are in control of your life and you demonstrate tremendous willpower over alcohol. You probably drink very little, as other areas of your life – family, friends, job – all have a higher priority than alcohol.

Once in a while you may over-indulge, but you quickly get yourself back on the right track as your health is very important. You are probably happy with your life, and have a great deal of energy to accomplish all that you want.

25–39 points: Caution! You may be becoming dependent on alcohol as a stress reliever. You may already recognize that things need to change and I would imagine you try to cut down, but then think 'Oh, just for tonight!' You may or may not want to cut down on your drinking, but cutting back could give you immediate health benefits at this stage.

24 points or less: Stop! Alcohol could cause heartache in your life. You know that you want to stop drinking, or drink very little – but you've never felt that you had it 'in you' to change. You have a general sense of being sick and tired of the lifestyle that you've been leading. You need to immediately quit drinking alcohol for at least a month in order to evaluate why you drink so much and get your life back.

Now, not all of you will have any problem with alcohol and will be slightly bamboozled by the inclusion of this quiz. I've printed it here to show how easy it is to get caught up in a drinking culture that will cause your weight to increase and your wellbeing to decline. A little alcohol here and there will do you no harm and probably do you some good, but when it takes over your life, it's time to rethink. The truth is that the need to give up alcohol stops many, many people from embarking on both healthy-eating plans and diets. If alcohol is your sticking point it really is time to work out why.

Ageing Before Your Time

Think about someone you know who drinks a bit too much. The chances are they look a bit puffy in the face and have bags under their eyes. Now consider someone who drinks *far* too much: they'll look much older than their years. Alcohol has a dehydrating effect on the body; when it becomes dehydrated, our cells compensate by retaining fluids. This results in enlarged blood vessels and bloating. Dehydration also leads to water retention as a result of impaired liver function, and that's where the puffy face comes from.

The Drop Zone Diet will have a significant impact not only on your shape, but your beauty. Cutting out alcohol and topping up your body with nutrient-rich, whole, fresh foods will make you look radiant and healthy. You'll literally shine from the inside out!

Best of All . . .

Alcohol wrecks sleep, disturbing its rhythm and interrupting sleep patterns. In fact, moderate alcohol consumption 30 to 60 minutes before going to sleep will help you to feel sedated and drowsy, and creates a slump in the brain chemicals that cause euphoria. However, once asleep, alcohol affects the restorative REM (rapid-eye movement) stage of sleep, which is absolutely crucial to health. Scientists at the sleep laboratory at the University of Chicago found that rats regularly deprived of REM sleep died within weeks. During this stage of the sleep cycle many parts of the body are healed and renewed; this is also the period in which hormones are released to control appetite and weight (see page 90).

When your 'sleep architecture' is interrupted by alcohol you feel it the next day. Poor sleep leads to increased fatigue and, when you feel tired, this is often when cravings kick in. What do you want? A sugar and caffeine (and maybe nicotine) boost! To get the best from the Drop Zone Diet, you'll need to conserve your energy by getting a good, restful night's sleep. And the very good news is that this diet is carefully designed to promote this type of sleep, not just because you've removed alcohol, but because it fills you with healthy, vibrant energy during the day that will leave you properly tired at night. What's more, you'll be relaxed and calm – the perfect precursor to a good night's rest. On the Drop Zone Diet you'll wake refreshed and raring to go. I guarantee it.

Start now . . . Slip into a warm (not hot) lavender bath, turn off the gadgets and the apps, bring out a good book, listen to a relaxation tape and then unwind. Let your body repair and replenish itself with the magnificently and wonderfully healthy foods you'll be eating. It won't be long before you wonder why you needed that wind-down or pick-me-up drink at all! Craving alcohol is just like any other craving – if you get the balance of your diet right, you won't feel the need for it.

Even when you have got to grips with your cravings for food and drink, you may be worried about another common problem: overeating. How will you survive on a very low calorie diet? How can you regain control of your appetite and your eating habits to feed your body *only* what it needs? Well, don't worry! We've got that covered and it's coming up next.

CHAPTER 6

The One Where We Stop You from Overeating

Having worked in the health and wellness industry for two decades, I know a thing or two about the hurdles that dieters face, and how people tend to feel when they are on a diet. For example, I know that most of you will be caught up in the food 'guilt trap': you eat something 'naughty' and then mentally beat yourself up for hours or even days afterwards! I know that most of you size up other people's food to see what they are eating, probably doing a calculation in your head to tot up the calories their meals contain, even though you are not the one eating the food!

Many (if not all) of you are utterly exhausted, not only with the quest to lose weight once and for all, but also with the mental fatigue that this daily battle brings. You probably have cupboards groaning with vitamin tablets (some out of date and still unopened), and most of you have no idea why you are taking them – apart from the fact that some magazine article said they would help you to lose weight/make you feel better/boost your energy . . .

You've probably got a host of plans for the 'new you', and plenty of ideas how to become that person, yet despite all this exertion, attention to detail and *huge* desire, somehow the changes you so desperately want haven't yet happened.

Let's get a few things clear:

- It's *not* normal to wake up exhausted after eight hours' sleep
- It's *not* normal to crave something sweet after a big dinner
- It's *not* normal to get an afternoon energy dip around 3pm each day
- It's *not* normal to rely on caffeine, sugar and cigarettes to get you through the day
- It's *not* normal to crave a glass of wine each night, just to help you unwind

It's very likely that this state of existence has become the norm for you, and you've actually forgotten how it feels to feel good! Once you've done the Drop Zone Diet, you'll experience something new and exciting:

- You will wake feeling refreshed every morning
- Your energy levels will shoot up
- Your will have constant, stable energy throughout the day
- You will sleep like a baby
- You will normalize your food intake *naturally,* without having to calculate calories or count points
- You will have clear, smooth, healthy skin

The benefits are countless. While on the Drop Zone Diet you will feel satisfied even though you are eating far, far less than you have probably ever eaten before. It can be a big psychological leap to believe that smaller portions of healthy foods can fill you up and give you the energy you need to operate at optimum level, and you may struggle a little at the outset, simply because your brain is refusing to accept this new regime.

Eating with your eyes

Paul McKenna, the author of *I Can Make You Thin*, did a fascinating experiment to prove the principle that we eat with our eyes rather than our stomach. He took six diners and gave them identical plates of food – an 'all-American breakfast', to be exact. Without exception, all six diners cleared their plates. The following day, the six diners returned and were given the same breakfast again, but this time they were blindfolded. On this occasion, the diners ate significantly less food – in some cases, less than 50 per cent of what was on the plate! Without a doubt this shows that we do eat with our eyes, finishing what is on our plates despite the messages coming from our bodies.

Less is Best

It is a *good* thing to eat significantly less food during the Drop Zone Diet. As a nation we have become gluttonous, eating to the point where we feel stuffed after most main meals. We even have to 'make room' for a little something else, so full are our tummies after the average meal. It's no wonder we've become used to overeating. We are surrounded by food, wrapped in tantalising paper or packaged to entice us when we are at our most hungry or vulnerable. Everywhere around us people are eating and drinking and it seems positively natural to join them – whether we are hungry or not!

When we overeat on a regular basis, we override our natural biochemistry – the ebb and flow of nutrients in and out of cells. We undermine the on/off signalling capacity of our hunger and appetite mechanisms, and we reach the stage where we misinterpret signals. For example, our bodies may be craving fluids, but we give them more food because we've misread the request. This gets worse over time.

As there is in all of nature, within your body there is a 'natural order'. Your body will thrive when the calories taken in equal the energy expended, and when the calories you take in are in alignment with your weight and body size. Overfeeding yourself throws out your body's natural order. Apart from everything else, the Drop Zone Diet will help you to claim that balance back again and allow you to become more in tune with your body's *actual* needs by giving you the opportunity to recognize its signals.

A tale of two hormones

The hormones leptin and grehlin help to regulate hunger pangs and hunger 'cessation' (in other words, the sensation of feeling full). They are manufactured in the body, and affect our brain chemistry. They have the ability to regulate appetite if they are treated well, making weight loss effortless. But you must be prepared to surrender control! Remember the exercises to help you be mindful (see page 27), and my suggestion that fluidity can help you to *yield*. Your body knows what it is doing, so let it work for you. To enable this to happen naturally, you must be still, quiet and unstressed enough to listen to your core physiological signals and messages. Leptin and grehlin will do the work for you, and help to bring your eating under control, so that it becomes natural and intuitive. Your body will guide you so that you eat only when you are genuinely hungry – and that you stop when you are full.

'When you don't get enough sleep, leptin levels are driven down, which leaves you less satisfied after you eat. Lack of sleep also causes grehlin levels to rise, stimulating your appetite so that you want to eat more – often at the moment that you wake.'

Grehlin stimulates appetite and gets you to eat when your body needs fuel. It's a fast-acting hormone that will tell you when your body requires calories for energy, rather than because you are bored or have a sugar slump. Leptin looks after your energy balance, suppressing the desire for food when you are full, which could be helpful to induce weight loss. Leptin connects with receptors in a region in the brain called the hypothalamus where it inhibits appetite. Coincidentally the hypothalamus is located within the limbic system of the brain known as the 'emotional brain', so this could be why there is such a strong emotional pull towards comfort eating when we are upset.

Working with, rather than in opposition to, these two hormones will take the pressure off *you*, and create more balance and control in the regulation of your natural biochemistry. When you begin to work in harmony with the natural physiological rhythm of your body you experience a sense of calm and peace. The longings and cravings disappear and are replaced with the knowledge that all is well. The rhythmic beat of your body is perfectly synchronized to the moment-to-moment shifts in circadian rhythms, as it is to the waxing and waning of the moon and the rise and fall of the sun. This may all sound a bit idealistic, but the message here is that stopping and considering *what* you are eating and *how much* can help these two hormones do their work efficiently and effectively. Here's what you can do:

- Involve yourself in your own food preparation and cook from scratch if you can

- Eat in silence as often as possible
- Turn off the laptop, TV and radio and put down your book or magazine. Just eat quietly and concentrate on what you are doing
- Keep your eating environment calm
- Eat plenty of colourful foods, to engage your senses
- Ensure that you chew your food well, enabling enzymes to break it down more easily, and thus send a message to the brain that you've got what you need
- Eat slowly and mindfully. Your body needs time to process the fact that your tummy is full; if you wolf down your food, you may have finished before it has even registered that you are eating!
- Be aware of portion control (in particular, consider how we eat with our eyes; see page 89)
- Be conscious that you are feeding and nourishing your body, not just eating for the sake of it
- Enjoy the connection between you and your beautiful body – much as a mother does when she feeds her child. You are nurturing your own 'inner child'

Eating is a wonderful process. Remember, nothing gets in your mouth without you putting it there. The Drop Zone Diet will support you in developing conscious eating. The foods are vibrant and colourful, and you will need to prepare them yourself. Although the portion sizes are very small because this is, after all, an extreme diet, you can still take the time to enjoy them when mealtimes roll round.

More tricks . . .

Listening to your body is important, but will that always stop you from overeating if you are hungry or suffering from cravings? On the Drop Zone Diet you will be satisfied and full, and a selection of small snacks will see you through periods where you need a little more. Eating extremely small meals on this diet will help you to adjust your mindset and realize that you simply don't need as much food as you thought you did. If you do feel hungry, try to get to the root of the feeling. Ask yourself: Am I really hungry or do I just want to change the way I feel?

We overeat for many reasons, including:

- Boredom
- Emotional or comfort eating
- Fatigue
- Social obligations
- Failing to be 'mindful' (in other words, eating while watching TV or reading, and not noticing what we take in)
- To fill a void
- Addiction

The next time you feel a hunger pang, ask yourself what's *really* going on. Assess your emotional state and what's happening at the time. Wait 15 minutes before eating anything at all to see if the feeling passes, and then drink a cup of warm herbal tea or hot water with lemon juice to soothe and restore you. Once you break the cycle of overeating for the wrong reasons, it's that much easier to lose weight and keep it off!

So How Much Do You Have to Lose?

One of the *very* best ways to ensure that you don't overeat is to have a clear-cut weight-loss goal. If your goals are vague and hard to monitor, you may not be as motivated to continue. The concept behind the Drop Zone Diet is not just to promote extremely quick weight loss to kick-start a new regime and get you back into those jeans with a boost of much-needed confidence, but also a way to begin to eat healthily and to experience the benefits of vibrant, nourishing food. As you begin to feel better on every level, you simply won't *want* to eat as much and you'll have every reason to say 'no' to that extra-large portion.

Setting a sensible weight-loss target is key to your ultimate success. Aiming for size zero if you are currently 12 stone will probably end in disaster, as your goal is incompatible with healthy eating. The ultimate aim of every diet should be overall health, and that naturally involves attaining and maintaining a *healthy* weight.

Height/weight ratio

The following 'ideal weight' chart is suitable for people who are 18 or over. It allows you to plot your weight in stones against your height, to see where you fall in terms of a healthy weight. Are you underweight? Are you obese? This system was originally designed by an insurance company to identify people who might be at risk of ill health in the future, thus enabling them to set an appropriate cost for health insurance. This graph provides an easy visual aid, which can help you to chart your progress once you have established your goal. Remember, however, that it is a guide only, as it doesn't take into consideration the differences in our frames and even in genetics. Only you will know when you feel in peak condition, and it may be at a weight that is just below or above what is considered normal here.

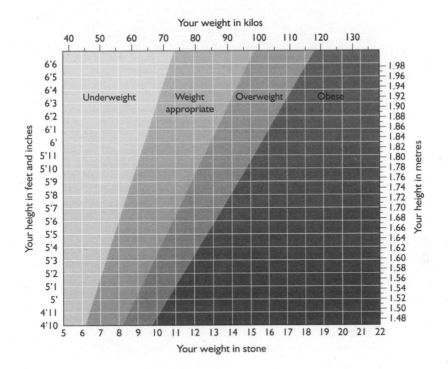

Body mass index (BMI)

A person's BMI is calculated by dividing their weight in kilograms by the square of their height in metres. This is one of the most commonly used ways of assessing an individual's healthy weight; however, it is, again, still just a rough guideline. It does not measure the percentage of body fat (in particular, the dangerous 'visceral fat' in the abdominal cavity and around internal organs), or account for the distribution of body fat. As you know, too, muscle weighs more than fat so potentially you could be very fit and healthy and still appear to fall into the overweight category. Once again, aim for a weight where you look and feel good, and operate at optimal level.

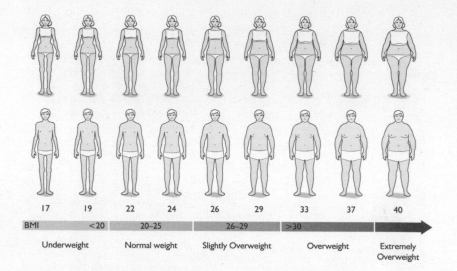

BMI	<20	20–25	26–29	>30	
	Underweight	Normal weight	Slightly Overweight	Overweight	Extremely Overweight

17   19   22   24   26   29   33   37   40

Waist circumference

A very quick health test you can do right now is to measure your waist circumference. A measurement of over 35 inches (89cm) for women and over 40 inches (102cm) for men means that you are at a much higher risk of developing health problems such as diabetes and cardiovascular disease, both of which are linked to excess fat in the diet and overeating. If you fall into the danger zone, you may well be instantly motivated to do something about your weight, and the Drop Zone Diet is the perfect place to start.

A short-term goal – in this case, 14 pounds in 14 days – can be useful as a first step. Once that's achieved, you can set another goal, and then another, until you find the weight where you are fit, healthy and happy.

Right now there is probably only one thing that is preventing you from achieving your ultimate goal of attaining an amazing body, and that's your brain. Negative self-talk can have devastating consequences and prevent you from losing the weight you want. It can lock you in a cycle of *wanting* to change but never finding the confidence to fulfil your full potential.

For that reason, let's go and put you in charge of your brain!

CHAPTER 7

The One Where We Build You a Brighter Brain

You might not want a fat body but you definitely want a fat head! About two-thirds of the brain is composed of fat – fats that give form, shape and structure to the brain, and allow messages to cross the membranes. For signals to be efficiently transmitted, the composition of your brain cells needs to have the perfect combination of fats. What does this have to do with your diet, I hear you wonder? One of the problems with rapid weight loss – and, indeed, crash diets – is that the brain can be effectively starved of essential fats. That's one of the reasons why you can feel forgetful, groggy or even confused when you diet. What's more, the brain also controls our emotions and the way we think. If it's not being properly nourished, we can become snappy, tearful and irritable; we can also lack motivation and willpower because our brains will tell us to give in to temptation and cravings in order to get some much-needed nutrition. The Drop Zone Diet, along with an important selection of supplements, offers key fats required by the brain, thus aiding its function, your weight loss and the ultimate success of your diet. In a nutshell, this diet will help you to feel great at brain level.

Essential Fatty Acids (EFAs)

As their name suggests, these fats are essential to health but they cannot be manufactured by the body and must come directly from the food you eat. Symptoms of EFA deficiency include:

- Poor memory
- Depression
- Dry skin
- Fatigue
- Poor circulation
- Eczema
- Excessive hair loss

EFAs are essential for the brain, helping to make up its mass and ensuring that messages are efficiently passed between its cells. In fact, your brain cells are formed from the EFAs you eat in your diet. That's one of the reasons why you feel so fantastic on the Drop Zone Diet: it's packed with the healthy fats that make up your brain cells. In particular, these are the omega oils (usually known as omega 3, omega 6 and omega 9) that are found in avocados, nuts, coldwater fish (such as salmon and mackerel), flaxseeds, hemp seeds, pumpkin seeds, sunflower seeds and leafy green vegetables. Without omega-3 fatty acids, brain cells stiffen and inhibit the messages that pass between neurons. Shortages of these oils have also been linked to low intelligence, learning deficiencies and depression. What's more, omega oils enhance cognitive, aural and optic development, which continue throughout life.

And there's more! Have you ever heard of prostaglandins? These are very specialized hormones that help to regulate blood clotting, body temperature, blood pressure, reproduction and even immunity. They are formed from EFAs by our body, but we also need certain vitamins and minerals to enable them to do so. These include vitamins B3, B6 and C, and the minerals magnesium and iron. Good sources of vitamin C include fresh fruit and vegetables, and you'll get iron from leafy green vegetables, meat, dried apricots, sesame and pumpkin seeds, whole grains and nuts. The Drop Zone Diet is bursting with B vitamins and magnesium (found in whole grains, pulses, nuts and vegetables). Are you starting to see why this diet is so effective?

Phospholipids

The predominant fats within the brain are phospholipids, which are made from a combination of fats and phosphorous. Two of the most important phospholipid components of brain cells are the fats phosphatidylserine and phosphatidylcholine. How's that for a mouthful? Both fats are crucial to brain function and thus your ability to learn, memorize, recall, feel awake and alert, and operate cognitively. Phosphatidylcholine, the most abundant fat in the brain, is also known as lecithin, and it's found in a variety of different foods including liver, eggs, wheat germ, soya and peanuts. Including these foods in your diet can improve brain health on all levels. You can also take a lecithin supplement (see page 124).

Brighter Brain, Brighter You

How's your focus of attention lately? Do you ever start reading something only to find that although your eyes are travelling across the page, the information isn't being retained or processed and you have to start from the beginning again after a few lines?

So many people are reporting that their memory, concentration and attention span isn't as good as it used to be and that they struggle to cut out distractions for long enough to fully absorb information – and retain it. It's like adult ADHD! Adult attention deficit hyperactivity disorder: an inability to quieten the mind for long enough to sit still and be peaceful without distracting ourselves with thoughts and images that aren't necessary at that particular moment in time.

Well, you now have a clear goal – a goal that will require absolute focus and dedication if you are to lose 14 pounds in 14 days. Your ability to concentrate and stay focused is paramount to the success of the Drop Zone Diet and now you have the information you need about the right fats, you can rest assured that these health-critical foods are contained within the foods on the diet to help you:

- Improve your memory
- Experience better memory recall (no more walking into rooms and forgetting what you went in for)
- Concentrate better
- Balance your moods

Gut instinct

It's your brain, not your stomach, that's hungry! Hunger starts first in the brain, due to low levels of the hormone leptin, which governs our balance of energy. The brain sends a message to the vagus nerve in the gut, and that's when we experience the sensation of hunger.

Putting You in Charge of Your Brighter Brain

Tucked deep in a crevice of your brain is your very own success tool kit! This is an area known as the reticular activating system (RAS) and you need to familiarize yourself with it for the duration of this diet (and beyond) because your RAS is unique to you. It holds the blueprint for the way you think, and its operations are actually one of the reasons why thin people stay thin and fat people stay fat. Thin people don't struggle to avoid cakes and biscuits, because they don't even *see* them! Fat people see glistening iced buns and delicious hot, salted chips wherever they turn. Why is this? Because their RAS operates this way. If you can get to know your own RAS and train it up, you will hold the key to easy, effortless weight loss. Here's how.

Your RAS is a network of fibres and cells that receives input via your central nervous system. It registers everything that your senses pick up, including what you see, hear, smell and touch. Your RAS only allows information that is pertinent to you to filter through to your brain – otherwise you'd have a barrage of stimuli that would probably send you mad! It filters out unnecessary information from the millions of signals your brain receives and focuses in on what you subconsciously want to register. It's a little like a magnifying glass, which encourages you to notice the minutiae of certain things that other people might not even notice, because their RAS is focused on something else.

I have a friend who is a policeman, and he has often mentioned that individual witnesses to the same incident all apparently see something different. Everyone picks up different things according to what their RAS has registered as being important.

Our brains also work on autopilot much of the time, simplifying things so that we can get from A to B in the best possible way. It will look for similar situations in the past – conclusions you've successfully drawn before – and it will use them, mainly because it likes order and repetition. The downside of this, of course, is that it remembers bad habits as well as good ones! So, if you've felt hungry in the past and you've satisfied that hunger with unhealthy foods like cakes and buns, experiencing pleasure at the same time, your brain will receive a powerful message right there in the pleasure centres! It will conclude that eating these foods is a good solution to hunger, and when you next become hungry you will be drawn to them. In fact, that may be all you see, smell and sense! Your brain has its very own filing cabinet with information that is valuable only to you. It gets worse! Chemicals called neurotransmitters strengthen the associations made by your brain. For example, compounds in chocolate initiate the release of dopamine, a neurotransmitter that provides feelings of elation and pleasure. Your brain connects chocolate to pleasure!

So it's time to do a little reprogramming. Any food can potentially bring you pleasure and satisfy your hunger. A chicken salad, for example, can also initiate the release of dopamine if you program your brain to think that way. The next time you eat chicken salad, really focus on how delicious it is – how good it makes you feel, and how it is *exactly* what you needed to make you feel great. *Mmmm*, chicken salad! *Mmmm*, crudités with hummus! *Mmmm*, fresh fruit smoothie! Get the picture? Soon enough your brain will start to notice these foods and draw them to your attention – at the expense of unhealthy options. Then you are nearly there!

Eating what you see

An American research team headed by Dr Brian Wansink looked at how visual mechanisms and environment influence appetite and the volume of food consumed. His team rigged up some soup bowls with pipes connected beneath the table to constantly refill the bowls as people ate. Some people ate from regular soup bowls and others from the 'rigged' bowls. The people in the latter category consumed, on average, 75 per cent more soup – yet didn't think they had eaten more than a bowlful!

Tricking your triune brain

It gets more complicated from here. Scientists call our brain the 'triune brain' because it is composed of three distinct parts. As we evolved, it grew from the bottom up in three stages that produced its three separate parts. These are: the reptilian brain, the limbic system and the executive brain. Whenever you have a 'mental battle' (for example, whether to eat a biscuit or not), there is literally a battle between each of these three parts of your brain.

Your reptilian brain is the oldest part of your brain: this is the one that would be likely to desire the biscuit and tempt you to eat it. It's concerned with our survival and knows that we need energy to survive. It wants you to consume calories (the biscuit) for energy. The newest part of the brain is the executive brain, also known as the pre-frontal cortex. This part of the brain is concerned with goal setting, and would probably be saying: 'No, I will not eat the biscuit, I'm on a diet and I'm sticking to it.'

The challenge comes when the limbic system gets involved, as this is the emotional part of the brain. In this case, it would side with the reptilian brain and say: 'Go on, just one! You know you're tired and stressed, and that biscuit would taste so good!'

You can take control of these warring factions and get them to work for you by setting a goal *firmly* in your executive brain, which will override any other messages. You'll need to be present and firmly conscious when you are setting the goal. If you are 'dual functioning' (for example, driving the car or watching TV), your goals will be diluted and that much less effective. Sit down quietly, gather yourself together mentally (all those bits of you that are still scattered at work or in the kitchen or worrying about your kids), and then ask yourself a question, such as, 'Where am I now?' This brings your executive brain into sharp focus, as it is a cognitive question that it wants to answer. When you have its attention, set your goal or goals. Do this every day for 21 days to reinforce the process (psychologists claim that it takes just 21 days for a new habit to imbed itself in our psyche). What do you have to lose?

Feeding your brain and training it to work for you are just two of the tools that can help to make the Drop Zone Diet a success – and also help you to feel fantastic while you are on it. After you've finished your 14 days on the Drop Zone Diet, ensure you continue to imbed your goals in your executive brain, and to train up your RAS to notice the things you *want* it to notice. With stable moods, improved memory and greater concentration you will experience more powerful willpower, the determination to continue right to the end – and once there to stay there!

You've got your brain in gear and you are now in charge of it, so it's time to get the rest of you moving. Not only will a little exercise get your juices flowing, increase your rate of weight loss and tighten up some of the wobbly bits, but it will elevate your mood, improve your sleep and help you to look better than ever before. It's easy, I promise!

CHAPTER 8

The One Where We Get You Moving

Wanting to change requires passion, desire and inspiration. The Drop Zone Diet is like gently shaking a snow globe – your stagnant energy will start to flow, allowing you the perfect conditions to let go of any negativity and create a new approach to health and nutrition. You will shop differently and buy healthier foods. You will cook differently, preparing foods from scratch as often as you can, and make more conscious choices around your health and lifestyle.

A new way of life beckons, one that is vibrant and energized, and revolves around a healthy you. What are you going to do with this newfound energy and how are you going to keep it as a constant in your life? How easy will it be to slip right back to where you began? How many times have you started a diet? Or joined a gym? How many diet books have you bought? Most importantly, how many times have you given up before you've really even begun?

Wanting change is a significant factor in the success of any new venture. The desire has to be absolute and true. You have to want it above and beyond anything else, so that when the going gets tough you can stick with it. It may sound odd, but exercise can help to create the right mental conditions for change. Exercise encourages the release of endorphins, the feel-good hormones, and leaves you feeling invigorated and strengthened, both physically and emotionally. It aids the release of toxins that may have been making you feel unwell, and it pumps freshly oxygenated blood around your body, improving your skin, hair, brain activity and cardiovascular health.

To enable you to flourish throughout the Drop Zone Diet moderate exercise is highly recommended. I'm not talking about taking on a 20-kilometre hike or joining an advanced fitness class when you've been sedentary for years. Instead, we'll look at ways that exercise will benefit you, the types of exercise that will complement the Drop Zone Diet, and what you need to get the most from them.

You have to want it!

Robert Sapolsky, a professor of neuroscience at Stanford University in America, demonstrated that rats who were allowed to run voluntarily on a wheel showed a variety of health improvements, while those who were forced to run against their will experienced worse health. Extrapolating the main point from this, it's clear to see that if you are negative about exercise and view it as a chore, you simply won't experience the same benefits – and it could even be counterproductive.

Reducing Stress

One of the most important benefits of exercise is its ability to reduce stress by dispersing adrenaline. It is this hormone that causes the symptoms of stress that 'distress' us all – shaking, sleeplessness, irritability, low self-esteem and mood, headaches, muscle pain, tension, digestive complaints, forgetfulness, anxiety and much, much more. Stress can wear out your adrenal glands (see page 46), which can lead to cravings and blood-sugar problems and is one of the most common causes of people becoming overweight. Many of us choose food to try to counteract its effects. In fact, stress has an immediate effect on your shape, causing fat to be laid down on your abdomen (the 'fat around your middle' effect) that is the most dangerous for health, but also probably the least attractive. Who wants a muffin top?

Stress temporarily increases blood-sugar levels by reducing the uptake of glucose (sugar) into the cells. So while you are dashing around, physically and emotionally charged, you are living in an 'altered state', with artificially high blood-sugar levels to give you the energy you need to get through the 'crisis'. The challenge is that when adrenaline (and the stress hormone cortisol) falls, glucose is then absorbed back into your cells and you *crash*! I suspect that this crash is one of the reasons why we experience evening 'munchies' and, interestingly, the need to have something sweet in the early evening is one of the main reasons that people cite for ruining their diets and giving up too soon!

The lawyer

As a lawyer, the long hours and pressure of work mean that I often skip breakfast, have lunch (often a dry sandwich) at my desk and don't eat dinner until after 8pm. This is hardly conducive to a healthy lifestyle. Jeannette came to my company to present some 'stress and nutrition' seminars, and I took the opportunity to have a one-to-one consultation with her. It was the best money I've ever spent. I'd been trying to make adjustments to my eating patterns and had bought a range of expensive supplements in a desperate bid to feel better; in truth, however, I either forgot to take them or just shoved them all in at once and hoped for the best. Jeannette smoothed my path by advising me how and when to take them, and explaining which foods worked best for my body. She gave me the Drop Zone Diet to help me shed some of my excess weight. And I felt like a light had been switched on inside me – I felt colourful again from the inside. The difference was so dramatic that I changed my lifestyle completely. Now, I always have breakfast and walk away from my desk to have lunch. I may still manage only a quick bite, but it's a break and I now recognize the psychological lift that this can bring. Because the results were so quick, the Drop Zone Diet was instrumental in my long-term shift. It made me feel great – and want to keep on feeling great!

'I'm OK during the day when I'm at work and I have a routine. I eat healthily and it's never a problem; however, in the evenings, it's a nightmare! I desperately crave sugar, chocolate and crisps – anything to keep me going. I inevitably end up sending my guy to the shops for a treat, and bang go all of my good intentions.'

Stress addiction can also be a problem. If your life swings from one drama to the next and your pendulum never really establishes a healthy rhythm, it's possible that you have become dependent both physically and emotionally on the 'rush' that stress tends to bring. Is it possible to become addicted to the drama of your life? Of course, you don't like the side-effects, but pumping adrenaline might, in fact, be something you've grown used to and now need. Interestingly, the stress hormone cortisol is highly implicated in depression, so if you are feeling low or anxious, it may be that your addiction has swung out of control. Exercise is an efficient way to promote good sleep, ease mood swings and disperse the chemicals that enter your blood when you live a stressful life. You may be amazed by how much better you feel after exercising for just 15 minutes a day.

You're Worth It!

Regular physical exercise produces immense rewards. Ideally, you should exercise for at least 30 minutes three times a week to experience optimum benefits; however, on the Drop Zone Diet you'll probably end up doing a little less. During the 14 days of the diet you will be taking in very few calories and the huge number of nutrients contained within the menus will be working hard to facilitate healing within your body, so it's best not to exert your body greatly during this time. You'll be changing the way you think as your body changes, and it's quite a special, almost spiritual time. Even if you are feeling more energized than you have in ages, it's important not to overdo it. Soon you'll be able to reap the rewards of experiencing a renewed zest for life and feeling far more vigorous!

It is worth understanding how exercise improves your health. It can fall way down the list of priorities in our lives, simply because we are pressed for time and often feel tired and stressed. The irony is that exercise can improve *all* of these feelings and more, and provide you with the energy you need to continue. You only have to start!

You will:

- Build a strong healthy heart
- Control your body weight
- Lower your blood pressure
- Reduce excess body fat
- Decrease cholesterol levels
- Sleep more deeply
- Diminish your risk of acquiring Type 2 diabetes
- Develop strong bones
- Elevate your mood
- Enjoy better sex
- Boost your energy

Are you still not convinced? Well, how about this? Exercise actually works to *clean your blood*! It stimulates your lymphatic system, which runs parallel to your circulatory system to remove waste and ensure that your immune system works at its optimum level. The lymphatic system is comprised of a network of nodes, ducts, vessels and glands distributed all over your body (in particular, your neck, throat, breasts, groin and knees). It doesn't have its own pump, so it relies upon the circulatory system to keep it moving. The better your circulation, the better your lymphatic system works – and the more efficiently it drains. It's like pulling the plug on dirty bath water and letting it all drain out! So when you exercise, getting your heart pumping and your freshly oxygenated blood rushing around your body, you are also kick-starting your lymphatic system, which joins in the frenzy and works harder than ever. The more efficiently it works, the better able your body is to cleanse and purify your blood of bacteria and viruses, not to mention all of the waste products it produces. A 2005 study found that lymph (the fluid in the lymphatic system) increases two- to three-fold during exercise!

Boosting the Effects of the Drop Zone Diet

However gentle it may be, exercise is a crucial part of the Drop Zone Diet, not just because it helps to make your body healthier, but also because it encourages your metabolism to speed up and burn off the fat you so want to lose.

Your usual exercise levels and starting weight will help to determine the intensity of the exercise you choose; however, in general, gentle to moderate exercise is best for the reasons noted above. Exercise that falls neatly into this category includes:

- Walking briskly
- Aqua areobics
- Cycling (on flat terrain)
- Hiking
- Swimming
- Pilates
- Yoga
- Ballroom or salsa dancing
- Golf
- T'ai chi

The idea is to raise your heart rate to the point where you are breathing heavily but capable of talking.

Higher-intensity exercise should be avoided during the Drop Zone Diet, as your energy will be required elsewhere.

It may be that you are very fit and comfortable continuing with a regular jogging routine, but slow things down to conserve your energy. If at all possible, avoid:

- Jogging/running
- Tennis
- Zumba
- Football
- Rugby
- Martial arts
- Mountain biking
- Gymnastics
- Other forms of highly aerobic or high impact exercise – anything that makes you breathe too hard to speak.

Targeting the Fat

To help address stubborn fat in specific zones, it's a great idea to practise a series of abdominal (tummy) and gluteus (butt) exercises every day. They'll really help to tone the stubborn areas that the Drop Zone Diet is working well to address, such as saddle-bags and muffin tops. And in case you were unaware of this, it pays to know that muscle is a fat-burning factory! Every little bit of muscle that you can develop will do even more to help regulate your weight both now and in the future. These exercises are not essential to the diet, but they will have an amazing impact on muscle tone, which in turn helps you to look tighter and leaner; they also help to strengthen your muscles, too.

You don't need weights or aerobics classes; you don't even need to work terribly hard. Gentle, regular exercise stimulates the development of muscle and its healthy growth; anything that you do now to encourage that will reap rewards in the future.

This means doing very simple things like lying on a mat when you are watching TV, holding your hands under the small of your back, and gently lifting up your legs together. Hold them at 90 degrees (in other words, perpendicular to the floor) for about five seconds, and then let them go. Gentle sit-ups work well too; press the small of your back firmly against the floor (or your mat) and keep your knees nicely bent. Or try 'cycling' by lying flat on your back and raising one knee to your opposite elbow, returning it down and doing the same on the other side. These exercises will all gently tighten your abdominal muscles, and can be easily done in a few moments of spare time.

As for your butt, even squeezing and tightening the muscles will make a difference — wherever you are! Nice deep squats work on both your butt and your thigh muscles, and holding them when you are down low for five or 10 seconds will enhance the impact. Walking up stairs is great for your bottom, which is why exercising with a step has always been so popular and effective. If you have an old step lingering in a cupboard, why not bring it out? Five minutes of climbing on and off will shape your butt before you know it. For another easy exercise, try lying on your tummy on a mat, and then drawing up your elbows and knees so that you are in 'all-fours' position. Carefully lift one leg upwards, keeping your knee bent. Hold for 10 seconds when you hit the 'top' of your mobility, and then bring it down. Repeat with your other knee.

I have a set of fantastic ab & butt exercises that really tone these muscles and help you lose inches on my website (www.jeannettejackson.com) if you are in the mood to push yourself, but the truth is that while these exercises will undoubtedly *enhance* your weight loss and your shape, all forms of exercise will benefit you. In fact, I've had clients in wheelchairs who were completely unable to perform specific exercises, but did manage to *move* a little more each day.

What *is* important is getting your heart rate up for 15 minutes every day and working to burn off that fat. Once you've finished the Drop Zone Diet, you'll undoubtedly benefit from targeting the areas that worry you most; for now, however, concentrate on becoming the person you want to be – both inside and out. Relax and enjoy the process of transformation; let your energy levels and your determination dictate how you move forward to become the fittest and the healthiest you've ever been.

Don't Delay

Exercise may be something you've successfully avoided for years, but if you embrace the idea of doing just 15 minutes every day, you will truly notice a difference. Meet a friend and take a walk in the park; try out your local swimming baths and spend a little time getting your stroke back; walk your dog for a little longer and faster than usual; turn on your iPod and dance to your favourite songs; do a little marching on the spot and stretching while you catch a favourite TV show. Try out a yoga class or borrow a bike to pick up the paper from your shop. Try to be creative about fitting exercise into your life, particularly if you've fallen out of the habit of doing it regularly. Challenge yourself to find 15 minutes a day, and try to make it work. The chances are that you'll enjoy it so much that after your diet has concluded you'll want more and more. That's one addiction worth pursuing!

You'll breathe better, you'll sleep better, and you'll feel the energy surging around your body. Best of all, you may even live longer, too. Are you ready to go? You'll need to get a few things in place before you embark on your life-changing mission, and we'll sort that out now.

CHAPTER 9

The One Where We Get You Prepared

This diet will enable you to lose up to 14 pounds in just 14 days. It's an extreme diet for extreme circumstances – maybe you have a holiday, a wedding or a special date in the near future! It's also the perfect way to finally shift the weight you've struggled to shift for so long. You'll lose up to (and maybe even more than) 14 pounds and this weight loss, along with the vibrant good health that you will experience, will encourage you to continue towards your ultimate goal. The good news is that you can enjoy the Drop Zone Diet up to four times a year, so doing it even occasionally can get you back on track when you've hit a plateau or lost enthusiasm in your life. I do recommend that you see your doctor before embarking on the Drop Zone Diet more than once a year, just to get the all-clear that it's OK for you to continue.

The success of this diet involves following it to the letter. It is designed to work integrally, with appropriate fluids, foods and exercise, and you'll need to do it *exactly* as prescribed to experience the full benefits. It's tried and tested, and it's worked time and time again. It will definitely work for you, too!

The Right Frame of Mind

The next 14 days can either be a form of torture to be endured as you give up your favourite foods to stick to a rigid plan *or* you can sail through it, delighting in the nutritious soups, foods and smoothies and the rainbow of colours and tastes they present. You can welcome the opportunity to replenish and renew your system while the pounds drop off or you can feel deprived. I know what I'd choose!

I suggest that you get very clear about your true goal. I know it's ultimately losing 14 pounds *fast*, but it helps to think about *why* you want to lose weight and what a 'lighter' future brings. Visualize yourself looking fabulous in those new trousers, or imagine people saying, 'Wow, you look amazing!' at a forthcoming event or on holiday. See the images very clearly and hear the compliments loudly in your head. Keeping it loud and visual will help you to stay strong – and remind you why you are doing this!

One thing I know for sure is that your desire to lose weight has to be greater than your desire to stick with your old patterns. You will have to learn to override your old habits, but the Drop Zone Diet is the ideal way to achieve this.

The Drop Zone Diet is the healthiest 'diet' around, with no exceptions. Your energy will rocket, your life will feel richer, and you will feel more fulfilled and experience greater emotional strength and increased confidence. Best of all, you will shift up to 14 pounds in 14 days! Get prepared for a new lighter you!

Taking Responsibility

Success is easier to achieve and maintain when there is a system or a strategy in place. A strategy sharpens our focus, keeps us on track and gives us structure to provide us with stability – particularly when we start to wobble. High on the list of amazing feedback about the Drop Zone Diet is the fact that it is incredibly easy to follow, and because it is spelled out so clearly, and so well structured, it removes the stress of having to think about what you are going to eat and when. Everything is done for you. You simply need to learn how to make the simple, delicious meals and eat them at the right time.

But it's not just the diet itself that performs the magic. You will become involved in the process of shopping for and preparing fresh, delicious foods that absolutely radiate health and nutrition. You'll see first hand the impact these foods have on all levels of your health – including your moods and your energy levels – and begin to understand the subtleties of your body. As I mentioned earlier, many of us are so used to feeling under par, we've forgotten what feeling good really is! Another important aspect of this diet's success is the fact that you are in the driving seat. You are selecting and preparing good food, not taking a pill, a potion or a meal-replacement shake or packet; you won't be buying ready-made low-calorie or low-fat meals or even having meals delivered to your door. You will be caring for yourself, and exercising your own power to make a change. That's a very good thing.

I know you are busy and probably juggling a million different things in your life. I do, however, suspect that regardless of how time-pressed you are, you do find time to brush your teeth every day – and probably more than once! Healthy eating needs to become as automatic this – something you do for the good of your health and because it is a habit. You need to reach naturally for healthy foods because that's what's been wired into your central nervous system. Don't underestimate the importance of your executive brain and your RAS on this one (see pages 102, 104–5). You can absolutely train yourself to *notice* the things that are good for you, instead of the junk that used to tempt you.

The Drop Zone Diet is hugely effective for another reason, too. It helps you to establish a new rhythm and routine, which can be the catalyst for a new way of living – and the birth of brand-new, healthy habits. Research has found that we rotate, on average, 15 meals over the course of a month. That means we are buying and cooking the same food over and over again. We dash into the supermarket and buy the same things; we may delight in the simplicity of streamlining our lives in this way, but what a rut we've created for ourselves! We may not even *notice* the fresh, seasonal produce lining the aisles – and if we do we may not know what to do with it!

The truth is that you aren't losing 14 pounds simply to put it all back on again. You'll want to stay slim and even continue to lose more weight if you need to. Breaking bad habits and experiencing the benefits of high-quality, nutritious food is the start of that – hence the beauty of the Drop Zone Diet.

Advance Planning

First and foremost, get organized! You will need to shop for the food and buy a few supplements to help you achieve maximum success on the diet. The good news is the supplements to help you achieve this are available on my website, where you can also download a FREE shopping list to make life much easier for yourself. Go to www.jeannettejackson.com for full details and enter the code DZ33 to download the shopping list.

Next, look through the recipes, make a list and head out to the shops. It's a good idea to make the soups in advance and then freeze them in 200ml servings. Each recipe will make enough for six servings, so you'll have three for the diet itself and then three extra servings for when you've finished. Try to shop every three or four days to ensure that your produce is as fresh as possible. And don't forget the snacks! They aren't an integral part of the diet, but they are designed to keep you going if you get the nibbles. Keep them on hand so that you can avoid temptation!

You'll also need to buy in the supplements that accompany the diet. These are chosen to enhance the impact of the healthy food you eat, as well as stabilize energy and blood-sugar levels and to help feed your brain. You'll need:

Acidophilus

This 'healthy bacteria' works to encourage the healing of your gut and the healthy function of your digestive system, and also supports your immune system. Better known as a type of probiotic, acidophilus also improves the health of your liver, as everything absorbed from the intestines passes through the liver in order for harmful substances to be detoxified before the rest of the body is exposed to them. If your gut is working efficiently, your liver has less to do and waste and toxins are more effectively excreted. Stress, excess alcohol, antibiotics, junk food and too much sugar can all reduce our natural stores of 'healthy bacteria' and taking a supplement throughout the programme can help to restore good health where it's needed. Alcohol can act as a mild laxative, so if you drink a lot then remove alcohol altogether, it can affect bowel functions, so it's crucial to get good bacteria in your body to make sure you stay regular throughout the diet.

Chromium

This mineral is essential for many metabolic functions in our body. It encourages the action of insulin from the pancreas; in fact, without it, insulin simply wouldn't work. Chromium governs our glucose tolerance factor (GTF), which controls our blood sugar. You'll be taking chromium on the diet to keep blood sugar balanced so that you experience the benefit of natural, healthy carbohydrates and, through that, consistent energy levels. A recent study of overweight women found that chromium supplements reduced their overall food intake, hunger levels and cravings for fatty food. An earlier study found that chromium prevented severe carbohydrate cravings in people suffering from depression. You'll need 200ug per day.

EPA

EPA stands for eicosapentaenoic acid, and it is a full-fat fish oil with a host of benefits. We looked at the importance of essential fatty acids for the brain (see page 99), but they also play an important role in everything from the health of your skin, joints, hair and heart to your memory, hormone production, mood, energy levels, vision and circulation. The main reason why I suggest supplementing fats throughout the Drop Zone Diet is their ability to generate energy for you. You'll be popping an EPA capsule, which includes DHA (docosahexaenoic acid), into your body at 3pm every day, which will be converted into energy by your body to give you the boost you need to get home for dinner, without a takeaway en route! If vegetarian take 1,000mg of flaxseed oil each day at 3pm instead of fish oil.

Lecithin

This is one of the most abundant fats in the membranes of our cell. It accounts for 30 per cent of the 'dry weight' of our brains, and 17 per cent of the central nervous system. Quite apart from that, it helps to break down fats in the body and regulate the flow of nutrients into and waste out of our cells. Lecithin is also necessary for a healthy memory. It's naturally found in eggs (it's the substance that makes egg yolks yellow), soya beans and vegetables such as cauliflower and cabbage. Like EPA, lecithin will boost your energy levels and help to reduce fatigue. Taking lecithin is not crucial for the success of the diet – you only need to take this if you are prone to fatigue. Go to www.jeannette jackson.com for more details.

5-HTP

5-Hydroxytryptophan is a compound that is manufactured in the body from the amino acid tryptophan. It is necessary for the production of the neurotransmitter serotonin (which encourages balanced moods and a feeling of wellbeing) and the hormone melatonin (which regulates our hormones and governs our body clock, amongst other things). Supplements are key to the success of this diet both because they lift your mood (in much the same way as an antidepressant would), help to normalize your sleep patterns so that you sleep soundly and wake refreshed, and also aid weight loss by removing cravings for carbohydrates and making you feel more satisfied by less food. Take 100mg every night around 8pm, to help you to relax and sleep deeply.

Coenzyme Q10

Coenzyme Q10 is a naturally occurring compound found in every cell in the body. Also known as ubiquinone, it plays an important role at cellular level in the mitochondria – the part of the cell responsible for producing energy (see page 45). Our bodies can make ubiquinone; however, our ability to produce it declines with age. If you find that your energy levels aren't as high as expected, it may be that a Co-Q10 boost is just what you need. Again, Co-Q10 is not absolutely necessary on the diet, but if you feel the need for an energy boost, you can take 30mg daily.

The actress

I'm an actress and travel around the country staying in cheap hotels and B&Bs, and I can tell you that you don't get offered peach and mango smoothies for breakfast at a guesthouse. I have always really struggled to sustain any kind of healthy eating plan (often eating takeaways in the evening on the way home from a performance), and excess weight piled on. I did the Drop Zone Diet when I was in a play near a friend's house, where I could stay and cook my own food. What I loved most about the diet were the delicious soups, which I took with me to eat before the performances. The results were so amazing that I paid to see Jeannette privately. What I've learned is that although I may not be able to eat healthily 100 per cent of the time, I simply need to do what I can, *when* I can. I'd fallen into a pattern of not eating well when I was at home, as well as when I was working away, as

I often felt sluggish. Now, I make the best choices I can when I am working away, and really zap up the nutrition when I am at home. Even though I've lost all the weight I needed to lose, I still eat the soups regularly because I love them so much!

Top tips for diet success

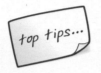

• Don't obsess about weighing yourself. Note down your weight at the beginning of the diet, on Day 7 and then on Day 14. It's natural to stabilize for a day or so around Days 8 and 9 as your metabolism aligns, and from a psychological point of view it's probably best that you don't see things slowing down.

• Do the ab & butt exercises that accompany the diet at www.jeannettejackson.com each day. They are an integral part of the plan, and only take 15 minutes a day. If you really can't manage them for health reasons, then walk, swim, dance or just shake to get your lymph and blood moving!

• Keep things to yourself. While some people like to broadcast their diet plans in order to gain support, you don't need to let everyone know that you are on yet *another* diet! I believe that dieting is actually a very personal process, as you are creating a massive shift within yourself. Get to know yourself on a different, peaceful level. It is quite a spiritual, sacred thing to have this time to evolve, so be gentle with yourself and show some self-respect.

• When you are finished, rejoice and tell the world!

Staying Hydrated

My university professor used to say that unless you switch off the 'dehydrate message' within the brain and bowels then everything else you do is effectively 'peeing against the wind'! It's a bit rude but it basically means what's the point of spending money on quality foods and oils if the body is too dry to fully appreciate – not to mention use – them? A dry body is arid and parched, and it under-functions on every level. Common symptoms of dehydration include:

- Chronic tiredness
- Aching joints
- Erratic pains throughout your body
- Irritability
- Poor sleep
- Constipation
- Wind
- Indigestion
- Dry skin
- Headaches
- Dizziness when standing up
- Poor concentration
- Confusion
- Fatigue
- Itchy skin
- Lethargy

Many of these symptoms will leave you feeling so under par, you'll feel depressed, moody and probably in need of some comfort food. Keeping your fluid levels topped up can aid your Drop Zone Diet success, and refresh you. It's rather like having an oil change to pep you up!

For optimum results, it is imperative that you drink approximately 1.5 to 2 litres of water every day – ideally fresh, still, natural mineral water. Herbal teas are also fine (and you are allowed one small skinny decaf latte or one decaf cup of tea each day, too), as long as you keep the fluid coming in. Top yourself up regularly, drinking at roughly equal intervals throughout the day.

It can be dangerous to ingest too much water in one go, as it can increase your total blood volume significantly, over-burdening your circulatory system, including your heart and blood vessels. It also puts pressure on your kidneys, which are forced to flush excess water out of your body at speed, to regulate the composition of your body fluids.

If you struggle to drink water (I can't tell you how many excuses I've heard to explain why people don't drink it, including finding the taste boring and being too 'busy' to remember to drink), try to remember how important it is to your body. All of your body functions depend upon water, and drinking adequate amounts can help to ensure the success of the Drop Zone Diet by keeping you energized, alert and even-tempered. Water also helps to flush out all the toxins that are released with your weight loss, and you'll feel lighter and brighter the moment they are gone.

Put it this way. If you had an ill goldfish, what would be the first thing you'd do? Change the water. A small change, but a big difference.

Liquid magic

- Start each morning with by sipping a large drink made from the fresh juice of half a lemon and half a lime. Give the fruits a good squeeze to extract as much juice as you can, then stir together with 400ml of hot water.

• Drink roughly 2 litres of water throughout the day.

• Herbal teas and one small skinny latte or cup of decaf tea will add to your fluid intake.

• No alcohol is allowed, no matter what (see page 74).

Super snacks

Each morning prepare **one** of these snacks to take out and about with you. Only eat it if you are tempted to grab something not on the programme.

- 60g steamed mange tout, with fresh lemon juice squeezed over
- 60g steamed (or raw) broccoli, with fresh lemon juice squeezed over
- 1 boiled egg
- A handful of cherry tomatoes
- 2 slices of cantaloupe melon, cubed

How the Diet Works

In the next section of the book, you'll find everything you need to create three delicious meals each day. There is a set meal plan for every day, but it is perfectly acceptable to move the days around to suit your tastes and even swap lunch for dinner or the reverse, if that works better for you. If there is a food you absolutely cannot stomach, you can repeat a meal you do like, as all of the foods are designed to work integrally, to help you lose weight quickly and easily. There are vegetarian options for all of the fish, meat and dairy dishes, so look for these if you don't eat meat or dairy or you want a change from the meals listed on the plan. It does help to be organized, making your soups in advance and ensuring you have all of the ingredients for all of your meals to hand.

There is a recipe for every meal, and also key notes on the health benefits of the foods you will be eating on each day of the plan. If you need a little motivation, it may help to remind yourself that you are improving your health and well-being as the pounds drop off, leaving you looking brighter, healthier and more beautiful as each day passes!

Try to start the diet when you have a quiet social period coming up. Too many deviations off the plan will definitely affect the amount of weight you lose. If you do have to go off-piste (with a wedding or a business lunch, for example, where taking your own food won't work) choose the healthiest food on offer and eat only a little. Whatever you do, don't drink alcohol, as it will set you back enormously. The absolute key to the success of this plan is following it carefully, so return to it for your next meal – no matter what!

When first shown this diet plan, some people have complained that they don't like vegetable juice, and asked if there is anything that can be substituted. In fact, vegetable juices are one of the most important features of the diet, as they help to alkalize the blood and reduce acidity and toxicity within the body, thus encouraging easier, safer and simpler weight loss. Instead of feeling exhausted and hungry, as you normally would on a very low-calorie diet, you will feel energized and well. The juices are a major part of that. If at the outset you don't like the taste of the juices, drinking them cold and through a straw will help, and as the days pass your palate will change to the point that you may actually start to enjoy them.

Another question I am frequently asked is whether there are any acceptable 'cheats'. If you are feeling unusually hungry and the prescribed snacks (see page 129) aren't hitting the mark, you can choose a healthy snack from the cravings table on pages 61–2. For example, three Ryvita crispbreads spread with a very thin scraping of Nutella hazelnut spread makes a lovely night-time treat. Accompany with a large cup of hot chamomile tea and you'll sleep like a baby!

Natural health and vitality exudes from confident people and this diet will not only enrich your body, but it will enrich your life, too.

I applaud your desire to get healthy and fit, and wish you the greatest of success with the Drop Zone Diet. It's time to begin!

PART TWO
The Drop Zone Diet Plan

The One Where We Do the Diet

You've got all the tools you need to make the Drop Zone Diet a success, and it's now down to you to show discipline, dedication and determination to get the results you want. If there's one thing I know for sure, it's that your desire to lose weight has to be greater than your desire to stick to your old habits. This diet gives you the opportunity to override them, but you've got to want to do it! Your 14-day meal plan is laid out in an easy-to-follow format and you can see at a glance what you'll be eating each day. I'll outline your food intake day by day, with amazing information on the superfoods you'll be eating and the benefits you will experience from the nutrients they contain. If there's anything that will give you motivation to continue, it's this! By the end of the diet, you'll not just be slimmer, but healthier, more energetic and balanced, too. Following your daily plans are recipes for each and every meal on the diet. Look at these carefully before you begin, to ensure that you have everything you need to create them to hand.

The beauty of the Drop Zone Diet – and why it works so wonderfully well – is that it offers a multifaceted approach. While you trim down the calories you eat, the foods on the diet also help to break down fat, speeding up the process while feeding your liver to encourage maximum, efficient detoxification. The Drop Zone Diet offers weight loss, speed and health – all in one concise time frame. It expedites weight loss in the most natural way possible.

However, two weeks is two weeks and I'm very conscious that during that time you have to function – go to work, see friends, eat, sleep and generally get on with your life. So, how best to support you through this period? Well, when I designed the diet I made five assumptions based on my years of experience and these are that:

1. You've tried loads of diets and this time you want one that *works fast*
2. You need quick, delicious recipes (who has time to faff about with elaborate menus?)
3. You want a diet that is simple, straightforward and incredibly easy to follow
4. You expect to feel amazing and look fantastic throughout
5. You want yummy, tempting food

You'll be getting all of this in spades! What's more, you'll find healthy alternatives to satisfy unhealthy cravings, and a few key supplements to support you throughout the plan. All this will help to make your 14 days on the Drop Zone Diet a positive, achievable experience. What are you waiting for?

Menu Planner

Below you'll find a menu planner outlining what you'll eat on each of the 14 days on the Drop Zone Diet. Remember that you can choose a vegetarian option at any meal, and you can swap lunch for dinner – and the reverse – whenever you wish. It's also possible to replace something you really don't like with a meal you *do* like, but I would ask you to give each recipe a try. Opening your eyes to fresh new foods and food combinations is one of the aims of the diet – along with weight loss, of course! Snacks are listed on page 129, and can be eaten as required, but do bear in mind that the more you eat, the more calories you take in, and the harder you'll have to work to burn them off. The good news is that you shouldn't be hungry on this diet, as it's perfectly designed to meet your body's core needs.

One thing you'll notice is that there is *a lot* of soup! The diet is primarily based around four soups, and you'll eat each one about three times on consecutive days. This is so that you won't need to worry about cooking up the whole range at once. These soups underpin the nutritional structure of the Drop Zone Diet and you will see that all of them contain onions, leeks, celery and garlic – cheap and cheerful ingredients that you can find easily and may even have to hand. Onions, leeks and garlic contain a compound called allicin – a natural antibiotic that helps to encourage a healthy immune system. They also contain sulphur, which acts as a powerful detoxifier to boost liver function. These soups will help to keep you fighting fit throughout the diet, and their ability to speed up the detox process will ensure that you have amazing skin, bright eyes and look fantastic from Day 1.

Go to www.jeannettejackson.com for a FREE shopping list to make your life so much easier. Type in the code DZ33 when requested for an instant download.

14-Day Menu Planner

Menu week 1

Day 1	Day 2	Day 3	Day 4	Day 5	Day 6	Day 7
9am: Take acidophilus capsule (look out for one that has a minimum of a million bacteria) each day at this time to encourage healthy 'gut bacteria', which helps detoxification, healthy digestion and the elimination of waste						
Carrot, Apple & Ginger Juice	Celery, Cucumber & Spinach Juice	Summer Fruits Juice	Banana Melt	Pepper, Broccoli & Ginger Juice	Avocado High-energy Drink	Orange & Pomegranate Juice
11am: Take chromium supplement (200ug) each day at this time to balance blood sugars and reduce the need to snack mid-morning						
Avocado & Rice Cakes	Tomato, Adzuki Bean & Chilli Soup with Rice Cakes	Avocado & Rice Cakes	Carrot & Ginger Soup with Brown Rice and Rice Cakes	Avocado & Rice Cakes	Carrot & Ginger Soup with Brown Rice and Rice Cakes	Lymph & Liver Tonic Cleanse
3pm: Take EPA/DHA pure fish oil (1,100mg) each day at this to time to boost brain power for the afternoon and provide energy to get you through to dinnertime						
Tomato, Adzuki & Chilli Bean Soup with Adzuki Beans	Cod with Green Beans & Courgettes	Tomato, Adzuki Bean & Chilli Soup with Adzuki Beans	Salmon with Corn on the Cob	Carrot & Ginger Soup with Brown Rice Adzuki Beans	Egg-white Omelette with Tomatoes, Mushrooms & Walnuts	Banana & Honey Delight
7pm: Take 5-HTP (100mg) each day at this time to encourage relaxation and restful sleep						

Menu week 2

Day 8	Day 9	Day 10	Day 11	Day 12	Day 13	Day 14
9am: Take acidophilus capsule (look out for one that has a minimum of a million bacteria) each day at this time to encourage healthy 'gut bacteria', which helps detoxification, healthy digestion and the elimination of waste						
Cucumber, Celery & Ginger Juice	Mango Smoothie	Watercress & Carrot Juice	Summer Fruits Juice	Beetroot, Cucumber & Ginger Juice	Carrot, Apple & Ginger Juice	Pineapple & Melon Medley
11am: Take chromium supplement (200ug) each day at this time to balance blood sugars and reduce the need to snack mid-morning						
Butternut Squash & Cumin Soup with Toasted Pumpkin Seeds and Black-eyed Beans with Rice Cakes	Avocado & Rice Cakes	Butternut Squash & Cumin Soup with Toasted Pumpkin Seeds and Black-eyed Beans with Rice Cakes	Avocado & Rice Cakes	Spinach & Nutmeg Soup with Quinoa and Butter Beans with Rice Cakes	Lymph & Liver Tonic Cleanse	Lymph & Liver Tonic Cleanse
3pm: Take EPA/DHA pure fish oil (1,100mg) each day at this to time to boost brain power for the afternoon and provide energy to get you through dinnertime						
Egg & Prawns with Fresh Greens	Butternut Squash & Cumin Soup with Toasted Pumpkin Seeds and Black-eyed Beans with extra Black-eyed Beans	Grilled Turkey with Tomatoes & Mushrooms	Spinach & Nutmeg Soup with Quinoa and Butter Beans with Borlotti Beans	Prawn, Asparagus & Spinach Salad	Spinach & Nutmeg Soup with Quinoa and Butter Beans with Borlotti Beans	Avocado High-energy Drink
7pm: Take 5-HTP (100mg) each day at this time to encourage relaxation and restful sleep						

Supplements available from www.jeannettejackson.com, where you can also download a FREE shopping list (download code DZ33)

Day 1

Breakfast:
Carrot, apple & ginger juice (page 171)

Lunch:
Avocado & rice cakes (see page 182)

Dinner:
Tomato, adzuki bean & chilli soup (see page 177) with added adzuki beans

Nutrition Notes

Carrot	Contains falcarinol, an anti-cancer compound, natural pesticide and antioxidant
Apple	Contains fibre in the form of pectin, which aids digestion, and polyphenols which help to lower cholesterol to improve heart health
Ginger	Alleviates symptoms of gastrointestinal distress and reduces inflammation
Avocado	High in vitamin E, a powerful antioxidant that helps to combat premature ageing, including wrinkling of the skin
Tomato	Rich in lycopene, a powerful antioxidant that is believed to help prevent a variety of diseases, including cancer and heart disease
Chilli	Helps to prevent hardening of the arteries and therefore reduce the risk of heart disease
Adzuki beans	Rich in iron, which is required by red blood cells for energy

Today's Superfood

Avocado

Avocado is the food of the gods and that is one of the reasons why it features so heavily in the Drop Zone Diet. Even if you don't like the taste or texture, I must urge you to do everything you can to include it. Over time, you'll not only become used to the taste, but even grow to enjoy it as your palate changes! It's an amazing food for skin, hair, nails and overall health.

What You Must Know A Healing Pod

Eating avocados can reduce the risk of heart disease. Avocados contain a mono-unsaturated fat, oleic acid, which is known to reduce cholesterol and inflammation in the body. It's nature's very own 'healing pod'.

What You Should Know Hand in Glove

Adding avocados or avocado oil to salads helps the body to maximize the absorption of the vitamins and minerals they contain. Fats within the avocado act as a 'carrier' to assist uptake and transport of nutrients into your body. Like a hand in a glove, the fats and vitamins lock together and absorption of key minerals and vitamins is greatly enhanced.

Nice to Know Makes You Thinner

People who regularly consume avocados are thinner than those who don't; they weigh less and tend to have a lower BMI. This is believed to be because healthy fats provide you with long-term energy and help you to feel fuller for longer. They may also help to suppress the appetite.

Day 2

Breakfast:
Celery, cucumber & spinach juice (see page 171)

Lunch:
Tomato, adzuki bean & chilli soup (see page 177)
with rice cakes

Dinner:
Cod with green beans & courgettes (see page 183)

Vegetarian option:
Pineapple & cashew nut sweet rice (see page 187)

Nutrition Notes

Celery	High in vitamin B2 (riboflavin), which helps to convert carbohydrates to energy
Cucumber	Helps to hydrate the body naturally and make fine lines in skin less visible
Spinach	Provides powerful antioxidant protection against heart disease and strokes
Ginger	Helps to reduce discomfort from stomach cramps and bowel distension, and reduces mid-afternoon bloating
Tomato	Contains chromium, a mineral that can help to regulate blood-sugar levels to reduce energy highs and lows
Cod	Fantastic source of low-fat, high-quality protein to help keep you fuller for longer
Green beans	Contain antioxidants that encourage cardiovascular health
Courgette	Contains omega-3 essential fatty acids, which encourage the health of your brain, skin and hair

Today's Superfood

Celery

The humble (oft called 'boring') celery stick is a super-food! It could be one of the main weapons in your armoury for successful weight loss and optimum health.

What You Must Know Lowers Blood Pressure
Celery contains compounds (phthalides) that help to relax the muscles around the walls of the arteries, allowing them to dilate. This creates more room for blood to flow freely around your body; the result is better circulation and reduced pressure on your heart.

What You Should Know Reduces Tumours
Other active compounds found in celery include acetylenics, which have a positive impact on the growth of tumour cells and may inhibit the continued growth and replication of cancerous cells.

Nice to Know Gets Rid of Puffy Eyes
Do you suffer from puffy eyes, or bags under the eyes? Celery is a natural diuretic that is rich in the electrolyte chemicals potassium and sodium – both of which help to regulate fluid balance in your body. Drinking celery juice for breakfast helps your body eliminate any excess fluids and helps your eyes look bright and refreshed.

Breakfast:
Summer fruits juice (see page 172)

Lunch:
Avocado & rice cakes (see page 182)

Dinner:
Tomato, adzuki bean & chilli soup (see page 177) with added adzuki beans

Nutrition Notes

Oranges	High in vitamin C, which promotes healthy bones, skin and blood vessels, including the delicate capillaries in the retina of your eye
Lime	Limes are excellent liver cleansers, and help to encourage the healthy flow of bile for digestion
Berries	Packed with powerful antioxidants to reduce damage to all cells throughout the body
Avocado	Contains glutathione, an extremely powerful antioxidant that binds itself to fat-soluble toxins such as alcohol, making them water soluble and easier for the body to excrete
Tomato	Rich in vitamin A, a fat-soluble vitamin that helps to improve night vision
Adzuki beans	Very low in saturated fats, sodium and cholesterol and a great source of protein

Today's Superfood

Berries
The ORAC (oxygen radical absorbance capacity) is a rating given to a food based on its antioxidant

content. All types of berries score exceptionally high in the ORAC league table, making them some of the most powerful antioxidants around. What does this mean? Antioxidants have a host of beneficial effects on the body, including protecting our cells from damage and disease, and promoting overall health. They've even been shown to slow down the degenerative effects of ageing, leaving you looking fresher and younger.

What You Must Know They Protect You Against Disease ✔
Polyphenol antioxidants in berries inhibit the oxidation of unhealthy 'LDL' fats.

In layman's terms, this means that they reduce the amount of damage that can be caused to the cells in your body, stabilizing free radicals (harmful oxygen molecules thought to cause damage to cells that can result in cancer, heart disease, arthritis and the process of ageing) and helping to escort them out of your body!

What You Should Know Helpful for Diabetes ✔
Berries have a beneficial effect on blood-sugar levels, too, according to the *British Journal of Nutrition*. Polyphenols in berries have been found to keep blood-sugar levels stable for longer, so less insulin is required by the body.

Nice to Know Blueberries to Go! ✔
You can freeze blueberries without damaging their ORAC capacity so there's no excuse not to eat healthily when you're in a rush. Keep a stock of blueberries in the freezer so you can add them to smoothies, porridge and even salads to give yourself a regular antioxidant boost!

Day 4

Breakfast:
Banana melt (see page 181)

Lunch:
Carrot & ginger soup with brown rice (page 178)
and rice cakes

Dinner:
Salmon with corn on the cob (see page 184)

Vegetarian Option:
Warm lemon & lentil salad (see page 187)

Nutrition Notes

Banana	Contains pectin which helps to soothe indigestion, heartburn and symptoms of an irritable bowel
Wholegrain pitta bread	A good source of protein, which is necessary for healthy hair, nails and skin
Honey	Raw honey has properties that help speed up tissue healing and encourage glowing skin, which is why it is often used in beauty products
Walnuts	Walnuts are a great source of omega-3 fats; eating just six to eight nuts will offer almost 100 per cent of your daily recommended intake. That's a huge boost for your brain, skin and hair health
Carrots	Chemicals contained within carrots have antibacterial and antifungal properties, which can help to restore imbalances in the gut and support the immune system
Salmon	High in omega-3 fats and perfect to replenish energy after a long day
Sweetcorn	Contains insoluble fibre that houses ferulic acid, an antioxidant that helps to fight diabetes and heart disease

Today's Superfood

Salmon

Salmon can either be farm-reared or caught wild from the sea, specifically from the Atlantic and Pacific oceans. The nutritional quality of salmon varies, depending upon where it's reared and caught, but salmon is always an excellent source of protein and healthy fats.

What You Must Know Boosts Brain Power ✓
Salmon is rich in omega-3 fats (essential fatty acids, or EFAs), which are an integral part of all cell membranes and crucial for cell formation and function. A diet deficient in omega-3 oils may cause the brain to age faster – and speed up memory loss. Omega oils are shown to help concentration and academic capability. This is because omega oils are integral to the manufacture of brain cell membranes, through which messages pass from cell to cell.

What You Should Know Can Reduce the Risk of Dementia ✓
Another fat found in salmon is DHA (docosahexaenoic acid), which is particularly important for the function of our central nervous system – and may even slow down the onset of age-related dementia. In fact, studies have found that people who eat two portions of oily fish every week show a 13 per cent lower rate of mental decline that those who do not.

Nice to Know Improve Your Memory ✓
Omega-3 oils help to manufacture a neurotransmitter called acetylcholine, which is involved in the renewal of brain cells, and required for learning and short-term memory.

Day 5

Breakfast:
Pepper, broccoli & ginger juice (see page 172)

Lunch:
Avocado & rice cakes (see page 182)

Dinner:
Carrot & ginger soup with brown rice (see page 178) and added adzuki beans

Nutrition Notes

Peppers	Contain the mineral molybdenum, which helps to breakdown uric acid, a by-product of protein metabolism, thereby improving detoxification
Broccoli	Like all members of the brassica family of vegetables, broccoli increases levels of glutathione, a key antioxidant that helps the liver get rid of toxins
Ginger	Its warming qualities promote healthy sweating, which assists detoxification and boosts immunity
Celery	Its alkaline properties make celery an important detoxifier, and chemicals contained within it encourage healthy digestion and assimilation of nutrients by the body
Avocado	One of the only plant sources that contains all 18 amino acids, which are the building blocks of protein, making it a perfect replacement for meat
Carrot	Chemicals contained within carrots have antibacterial and antifungal properties, which can help to restore imbalances in the gut and support the immune system
Adzuki beans	Valuable source of vegetable protein, which help to trim the waist while providing important amino acids to support your body

Today's Superfood

Broccoli

Broccoli has been eaten as a health food since Roman times; its edible florets and fibrous stalk provide numerous nutritional benefits. Plants absorb minerals from the soil and when we eat the plants we take on board the very minerals that help the plant to form and grow. Fable has it that broccoli was a staple food when Roman warriors known as legionaries prepared for war, because of its ability to provide strong bones and stamina.

What You Must Know High in Calcium

Broccoli is a good source of calcium for people who are dairy intolerant or have a vegan diet. Calcium protects against osteoporosis (brittle bone disease), but it needs vitamin K to move the calcium from our food to our bones. Broccoli is rich in both calcium and vitamin K, making it a fantastic addition to any diet.

What You Should Know Helps Combat Insomnia

Calcium in broccoli can also help to alleviate insomnia and promote a deep, restful night's sleep if eaten before bed, as it relaxes muscles, preventing spasms and cramps. Calcium can also help to reduce the risk of kidney stones in the body, as dietary calcium binds to waste products in the stomach called oxalates, and they are rapidly removed from the body along with any excess calcium.

Nice to Know Low-Calorie Snack

Broccoli is very low in calories, so its florets make superb crudités for snacking; just two raw or lightly steamed florets count as one of your 'five a day'.

Day 6

Breakfast:
Avocado high-energy drink (see page 173)

Lunch:
Carrot & ginger soup with brown rice (see page 178)
and rice cakes

Dinner:
Egg-white omelette with tomatoes, mushrooms &
walnuts (see page 184)

Vegetarian option:
Baked mushrooms with pine nuts (see page 188)

Nutrition Notes

Avocado	All proteins in avocado are readily digested and absorbed, thanks to the fibre it contains
Yoghurt	Yoghurt is easier to digest than cow's milk and therefore a great source of calcium for people who are lactose-intolerant
Lime	Limonoids, compounds found in both lemons and limes, have been shown to fight mouth cancer, skin cancer, lung cancer, breast cancer, stomach cancer and colon cancer
Carrot	Studies show that people who regularly eat carrots have lower incidence of glaucoma (a disease where the optic nerve is damaged by faulty pressure within the eyeball)
Egg	Contains sulphur, which assists the liver in the process of producing bile for efficient digestion
Mushroom	Fantastic for the immune system as it contains powerful polysaccharides that have strong antibacterial properties
Walnut	Contains an antioxidant known as ellagic acid, which supports the immune system and acts as an anti-cancer agent

Today's Superfood

Eggs

Eggs have caused such confusion in the health arena over the last few years in the 'Are they healthy?/Are they not?' debate. Well, the consensus amongst scientists and nutritionists (including me!) is that they are a wonderful, vital superfood that is essential for a healthy diet!

What Must You Know? Help Metabolic Health

Eggs are a good source of iodine, which is required for the manufacture of hormones essential for life, including thyroid hormones. Iodine is also required for the smooth running of the body's metabolism, which controls body temperature. An iodine deficiency presents as a goitre in the neck – a swelling of the thyroid gland that grows as the body accumulates white blood cells in the area.

What You Should Know Egg Yolks Protect Eye Health

Macular degeneration (MD) is an age-related, progressive disease of the retina in the eye and it affects sight in the centre of our field of vision. Eggs contain the nutrients lutein and zeaxanthin, which can help prevent this degeneration and support overall eye health.

Nice to Know Eggs Curb Your Hunger

Egg-based meals help people to feel fuller for longer. Scientists have discovered that people who eat eggs as opposed to a bagel for breakfast are less likely to need a mid-morning snack. Research found that they also consumed fewer calories over a 24-hour period than those who did not eat them.

Day 7

Breakfast:
Orange & pomegranate juice (see page 173)

Lunch:
Lymph & liver tonic cleanse (see page 183)

Dinner:
Banana & honey delight (see page 174)

Nutrition Notes

Oranges	With zero saturated fat or cholesterol, these are a fabulous source of immune-boosting vitamin C
Pomegranate	Rich in micronutrients, including potassium for nerve function, muscle control and healthy blood pressure
Grapefruit	Limonoids, the phytonutrients in grapefruit, prevent the formation of tumours by promoting the formation of an enzyme responsible for detoxification
Mange tout	High in fibre, which helps to maintain intestinal motility and also supports healthy cholesterol levels
Kale	Very rich in magnesium, which is vital for relaxing muscles and nerves, and building and strengthening bones
Lemon	Citrus fruits are rich in vitamin C, which is necessary for the manufacture of collagen for beautiful skin
Milk	Contains the amino acid tryptophan, which helps to manufacture serotonin (see page 124) when it is eaten alongside carbohydrates
Banana	An exceptionally rich source of fructo-oligosaccharide, a prebiotic that encourages the growth of healthy bacteria in the gut
Manuka honey	Contains powerful antibacterial properties beneficial for the health of the immune system
Pecans	A diet rich in nuts can reduce the risk of gallstones in women

Today's Superfood

Manuka honey

Manuka honey comes from bees that feast on the pollen of the Manuka bushes in New Zealand. It offers amazing health and healing properties, and there is some evidence that it may even be able to reverse resistance to antibiotics. Manuka honey has a 'UMF' (Unique Manuka Factor), which denotes the level of its antibacterial properties. Manuka honey with a UMF of 10 would be less powerful than one with a UMF of more than 20.

What You Must Know Fights Bacteria

The active antibacterial components in Manuka honey have been shown to reduce the impact of three bacteria (including the dreaded MRSA superbug) known to infect wounds by preventing bacteria from attaching to the wound tissue. Without bacteria the healing process will be maximized.

What You Should Know It's a Good Carb!

Unlike most other sweeteners, honey contains small amounts of a wide array of vitamins, minerals and amino acids, and is a great source of carbohydrates that place little stress on the digestive system, having been 'pre-digested' by bees.

Nice to Know Sshhh . . . Beauty Secret

I take Manuka honey every day as I adore the taste and I have personally found it boosts my energy and definitely contributes to my healthy hair and eyes.

Day 8

Breakfast:
Celery, cucumber & ginger juice (see page 174)

Lunch:
Butternut squash & cumin soup with toasted pumpkin seeds and black-eyed beans (see page 179) and rice cakes

Dinner:
Egg & prawns with fresh greens (see page 185)

Vegetarian option:
Healthy bean burrito (see page 189)

Nutrition Notes

Celery	Excellent source of dietary fibre, which helps support healthy bowels
Cucumber	High in phytonutrients called lignans that are known to have anti-cancer benefits
Ginger	Gingerols found in ginger have powerful anti-inflammatory properties
Butternut squash	Rich in complex carbohydrates to help maintain healthy blood-sugar levels
Eggs	Contain high levels of lecithin, which is a fat emulsifier (see page 124)
Prawns	Good source of tryptophan (see page 124) to help balance sleep and stabilize moods
Spinach	More than 23 different flavonoids have been discovered in spinach, which work as antioxidant and anti-cancer agents
Beetroot	Beetroot is rich in the antioxidant enzyme glutathione, which acts as the bodyguard for liver cells, protecting them from free-radical attack
Lemon	Restores the pH of your saliva, which helps you to absorb the nutrients from the food you eat

Today's Superfood

Ginger

Ginger root has been used for medicinal purposes for over 2,000 years, since it was first discovered in South East Asia. Raw ginger has been used to treat a variety of ailments, including heartburn, nausea and digestive problems.

What You Must Know Relieves Migraines

Ginger contains an active compound called gingerol, which is related to the chemical that gives chilli peppers their kick. Gingerol is said to have positive physiological effects for migraine sufferers, who have reported a reduction in the frequency of attacks when root ginger is taken as soon as the headache sets in.

What You Should Know Helps Motion Sickness

Ginger calms the digestive system and soothes the gut. It also stimulates the digestive enzymes, which makes it a traditional remedy still used today for travel sickness and even morning sickness during pregnancy.

Nice to Know Boosts Circulation

Do you always feel the cold? Ginger helps to warm the body and improve circulation, allowing the blood to flow more freely through your body and helping to prevent strokes.

Day 9

Breakfast:
Mango smoothie (see page 175)

Lunch:
Avocado & rice cakes (see page 182)

Dinner:
Butternut squash & cumin soup with toasted pumpkin seeds and black-eyed beans (see page 179) with added black-eyed beans

Nutrition Notes

Mango	Enzymes found in mango, including mangiferin, catechol oxidase and lactase, are excellent bowel cleaners
Yoghurt	Contains probiotics that reduce intestinal inflammation and fungal infections, and eliminate unhealthy bacteria that can damage the walls of the gut
Manuka honey	Contains phytonutrients (plant nutrients) that have been shown to have cancer-preventing and anti-tumour properties
Avocado	Contains manganese required for healthy skin, nails and hair
Butternut squash	Contains trace amounts of choline (a key component of brain cells) that can boost brain power
Black-eyed beans	High in antioxidant compounds called anthocyanins that protect many body systems

Today's Superfood

Mango

Mango is a luscious, sweet fruit with a fleshy pulp that can be enjoyed raw or cooked in chutneys, curries and sauces. Mangos are packed with vitamins and minerals that can help your body fight infection, reduce cholesterol levels and even improve your sex life!

What Must You Know? Excellent for De-stressing
Mango is rich in vitamin B6, the anti-stress vitamin. It's required to help you relax, deal with stress more efficiently, and also sleep more deeply, largely because it is required for the manufacture of the neurotransmitters GABA (which induces sleep, pain relief and relaxation) and serotonin (which regulates mood, sleep and appetite, amongst other things).

What You Should Know Helps to Clean the Bowels
Mango contains enzymes that help to purify the bowel, eliminating putrefying factors that make you feel tired and ill.

Nice to Know Have Better Sex!
Mango improves your sex life! It's high in vitamin E, which assists in the regulation of sex hormones in both men and women. It also helps in sperm production, so if things are a little slow on the conception front, this is the superfood for you!

Breakfast:
Watercress & carrot juice (see page 175)

Lunch:
Butternut squash & cumin soup with toasted pumpkin seeds and black-eyed beans (see page 179) and rice cakes

Dinner:
Grilled turkey with tomatoes & mushrooms (see page 186)

Vegetarian option:
Minted three-bean salad (see page 190)

Nutrition Notes

Watercress	Excellent for eye health as it contains the powerful carotenoids lutein and zeaxanthin
Carrot	Just one mugful of carrots supplies more than 600 times the suggested daily intake for vitamin A (in the form of beta carotene), one of the best antioxidants around
Lemon	Contains vitamin B5 (pantothenic acid) which helps to replenish the body in stressful times
Butternut squash	High in fibre, which helps to clear the intestine of waste for healthy bowel function
Turkey	Contains the amino acid tryptophan, which helps the brain to manufacture serotonin, the 'happy hormone', which helps you feel relaxed and peaceful; tryptophan also encourages restful sleep
Tomatoes	The carotenoids in tomatoes also encourage the production and activity of detoxification enzymes in the liver
Mushrooms	Contain good levels of iron, potassium, phosphorus, selenium, vitamin D and vitamin C, as well as protein and dietary fibre to keep you feeling great

Today's Superfood

Turkey
Not just for Christmas, turkey is an excellent form of protein that is also low in fat, making it a superb alternative to red meat. It's nutritious, with lots of iron in particular, and has been shown to keep blood-sugar levels steady for longer after meals, thus reducing the risk of Type 2 diabetes.

What You Must Know Lifts Depression
Turkey is high in the amino acid tryptophan, which enhances serotonin production in the brain, helping to relieve symptoms of depression and anxiety.

What You Should Know Boosts Your Immune System
Turkey contains good quantities of a trace mineral called selenium, which is required for a healthy immune system to defend against bacteria, viruses and other infections. Including turkey in your diet could help you ward off coughs and colds, and generally improve your health and wellness.

Nice to Know Stay Fuller for Longer
Turkey's high protein content bulks you up and makes you feel fuller for longer, thus helping you to lose weight without feeling hungry.

Breakfast:
Summer fruits juice (see page 172)

Lunch:
Avocado & rice cakes (see page 182)

Dinner:
Spinach & nutmeg soup with quinoa and butter beans (see page 180) with added borlotti beans

Nutrition Notes

Oranges	Vitamin C enhances liver function, which helps to clean the blood; it's also a key player in helping you to look glowing, fit and healthy
Lime	Excellent liver cleanser, helping to encourage the healthy flow of bile for digestion
Berries	Blueberries and raspberries contain lutein, which is essential for healthy eyesight; all berries contain fantastic antioxidants
Avocado	A source of carotenoids, such as zeaxanthin, which guard against inflammation
Spinach	A key ingredient of spinach is folate, necessary for healthy tissue throughout your body
Beans	Low in quick-release sugars to prevent blood-sugar spikes and energy dips
Quinoa	A seed not a grain, quinoa is one of the only plant foods to supply all of the essential amino acids for growth; it also contains high levels of omega-3 oils, to aid heart health and to give beautiful hair and skin

Today's Superfood

Spinach

Think spinach, think iron. It's probably the first thing that pops into people's heads when they think of this vegetable, but there's so much more to spinach than meets the eye. Green leafy vegetables are packed with antioxidants and scientists have discovered a positive link between these vegetables and halting the progression of prostate cancer. It is an excellent source of vitamin K, which is required for bone health (in fact, just one mugful of cooked spinach offers over 1,000 per cent of the daily recommended intake of this key vitamin), as well as double the recommended intake of beta-carotene.

What You Must Know Could Reduce the Risk of Cancer ✓
Inflammation is flagged up as a risk for the development of cancer and spinach contains chemicals that are known to reduce inflammation in all of our tissues.

What You Should Know Helps to Build Strong Bones ✓
Spinach is rich in a trio of nutrients, all of which help to ensure healthy bone formation. These nutrients include calcium, magnesium and vitamin K, which work in synergy to ensure optimum bone mass. They also work to reduce damage caused by infection.

Nice to Know Makes You Beautiful ✓
Spinach is jam-packed with antioxidants required for the manufacture of healthy cells, including those found in your hair, skin and nails. Beta-carotene is required for the growth and repair of body tissues, and this is one of the most abundant sources of this nutrient. Including spinach in your diet will help you to look luscious and fresh!

Day 12

Breakfast:
Beetroot, cucumber & ginger juice (see page 176)

Lunch:
Spinach & nutmeg soup with quinoa and butter beans (see page 180) with rice cakes

Dinner:
Prawn, asparagus and spinach salad (see page 186)

Vegetarian option:
Warm pumpkin & chickpea salad (see page 190)

Nutrition Notes

Beetroot	Bacteria in our saliva converts the nitrates in beetroot into nitric oxide, which is believed to reduce blood pressure
Cucumber	The high water content makes it an excellent source of hydration, while the vitamin C and caffeic acid help to prevent water retention
Ginger	Has proven antioxidant and anti-inflammatory effects
Butternut squash	High in beta-carotene that has countless health benefits, including guarding the skin against the harmful rays of the sun
Prawns	Low in calories and a good source of protein, prawns are a good source of omega oils that encourage heart health – not to mention skin and hair health
Spinach	When combined with fresh lemon, the iron in spinach can be accessed more efficiently by the body to boost energy levels
Tomato	Cooking tomatoes increases their lycopene content, which has been shown to provide powerful protection against cancer

Today's Superfood

Beetroot

Ah, beetroot, the Marmite of vegetables! You either love it or loathe it. I can tell you now that it's worth learning to love it, as the health benefits of this vibrant vegetable are unbelievable. Its vivid colour probably gives the game away – nothing this colourful could fail to be healthy!

What You Must Know Detox Magic ✓
The liver is the main organ of detoxification in the body and plays an important role in digestion and the breakdown of toxins. Beetroot is rich in the antioxidant enzyme gluta-thione, which is required by the liver to do its job. When you eat beetroot, you are helping your body to both break down and eliminate toxins easily, quickly and, above all, safely.

What You Should Know Helps to Keep Your Heart Strong ✓
Beetroot contains magnesium, an electrolyte mineral that is utilized in over 300 enzyme reactions within the body. It is required for healthy nerve and muscle function. The heart is one of the most important muscles in the body, and for that reason magnesium is crucial for optimum heart health.

Nice to Know Beetroot Cleans the Blood ✓
Beetroot juice has been shown to inhibit the formation of nitrosamine residues (carcinogenic chemicals that are the by-product of different foods we eat) in the stomach. Eating it regularly may help to prevent various cancers throughout the body.

Day 13

Breakfast:
Carrot, apple & ginger juice (see page 171)

Lunch:
Lymph & liver tonic cleanse (see page 183)

Dinner:
Spinach & nutmeg soup with quinoa and butter beans (see page 180) with added borlotti beans

Nutrition Notes

Carrot	The bright orange colour of carrots is caused by beta-carotene, a powerful antioxidant and a precursor to vitamin A
Apples	The pectin in apples acts as a binding agent bringing waste products together and ensuring they are eliminated from the body quickly and easily
Ginger	Aids the breakdown of proteins and fatty foods for smooth digestion
Grapefruit	Contains pectin, a soluble fibre that encourages healthy detoxification and lowers cholesterol, which can lead to clogged arteries
Mange tout	Provide a good mix of soluble and non-soluble fibre to aid and support healthy digestion and the elimination of waste from the body
Kale	Rich in glucosinolates, which can help to boost liver function
Lime	Can help to reduce excess body odour, due to its disinfectant effect
Spinach	Contains good levels of choline, one of the most abundant fats in the brain
Borlotti beans	High in potassium, to ensure good kidney function to excrete the toxins in urine

Today's Superfood

Apples

Delicious, juicy, readily available and inexpensive! Apples are a fantastic addition to any healthy diet as they contain a huge number of key nutrients required for overall health and wellbeing. They are the fruit richest in vitamin E, and contain good quantities of the B vitamins, biotin and folic acid, which are essential for energy and digestion. Apples also contain the antioxidant vitamins A and C, and more than 12 minerals.

What You Must Know An Apple a Day Reduces the Risk of Alzheimer's Disease

Scientists have found that mice fed on a regular diet of apple juice had higher levels of acetylcholine, a neurotransmitter required for healthy brain-to-cell nerve transmission. It's believed that the antioxidant quercetin, found in high levels in apples, is responsible. The mice fed on apple juice performed better on memory and cognitive tests than those who were not.

What You Should Know An Apple a Day Keeps Blood Clots at Bay

Apples contain rutin, a compound currently being investigated for its potential to prevent heart attacks and strokes. It seems that rutin can block the activity of a damaging enzyme called PDI (protein disulfide isomerase), which is released when blood clots form in arteries and veins. Rutin has proved to be effective in blocking the activity of this enzyme and could therefore be instrumental in reducing the risk of stroke.

Nice to Know Apple Cider Vinegar

Apple cider vinegar is made by crushing mature apples and allowing them to ferment. Consuming the fermented vinegar provides numerous potential health benefits, including reducing the incidence and duration of sinus infections and sore throats, and also helping to treat acne, fight allergies and prevent urinary tract infections. Best of all, apple cider vinegar has been shown in various studies to promote weight loss by impacting insulin secretion, preventing the accumulation of fat. It has been proved to have a beneficial impact on blood-sugar levels, and is currently being investigated as a form of treatment for Type 2 diabetes. There is also evidence that it can lower high cholesterol. Amazing!

Day 14

Breakfast:
Pineapple & melon medley (see page 182)

Lunch:
Lymph & liver tonic cleanse (see page 183)

Dinner:
Avocado high-energy drink (see page 173)

Nutrition Notes

Pineapple	Contains bromelain, a complex blend of chemicals, which includes protein-digesting enzymes, anti-inflammatory agents, anti-coagulants (natural blood-thinners) and overall help for the digestive system, including the colon and liver
Cantaloupe melon	Contains fat-soluble lycopene and beta-carotene and acts as an amazing diuretic to remove excess water from the body
Manuka honey	Excellent source of immediate energy for the body to boost blood-sugar levels and feed the brain
Grapefruit	Antiviral, antiseptic and diuretic properties, working specifically on the digestion and skin
Mange tout	Contains lutein, which helps to reduce the risk of macular degeneration of the eyes (see page 153) and cataracts
Kale	Contains a chemical called Indole-3-carbinol, which helps to balance menstrual cycles and process oestrogen
Lime	Flavonoids help to lower cholesterol
Avocado	Oleic acid found in avocados is known to assist heart health
Yoghurt	Contains good levels of calcium, potassium and magnesium, B vitamins and iodine (which encourages healthy thyroid function and metabolism)
Oranges	Contain limonene, which has the ability to inactivate toxins and encourage their excretion from the body
Lemon	Great source of vitamin B3 (niacin), which helps to reduce fatigue and depression

Today's Superfood

Pineapple

This delicious, versatile fruit can be enjoyed fresh, canned (in its own juice) grilled, barbecued or juiced and provides a wealth of vitamins and minerals. Eating is a sensory activity and the bright yellow flesh of this fruit is as invigorating to the eyes as it is to the palate. The high levels of vitamin C assist antioxidant production, and manganese and B vitamins (in particular thiamine) help to improve energy levels.

What You Must Know Helps to Soothe Indigestion and Wind ✓
Pineapple contains bromelain, an active plant enzyme also found in papayas. This enzyme, located in the stem of the pineapple, is known as a proteolytic enzyme because of its ability to digest proteins. A slice of pineapple with breakfast is said to stimulate digestive juices and enzymes to aid the digestion of food first thing in the morning. It's also a traditional remedy for heartburn – particularly during pregnancy.

What You Should Know Soothes Sinus Inflammation ✓
Bromelain has anti-inflammatory properties and can help to reduce swelling in cavities such the sinuses and nasal passages. It is also said to be very useful for sore throats.

Nice to Know Makes Your Eyes Bright and White ✓
Pineapple has a water content of 87 per cent, and it also contains good levels of the mineral potassium. Together, these create the positive effect of counteracting the negative effects of high levels of salt within the body, as well as helping to flush out unwanted toxins and acids, giving you a bright-eyed, healthy glow.

RECIPES

All of the meals in the Drop Zone Diet are easy to prepare and based on fresh, nutritious ingredients. All of the recipes serve one, apart from the soups which are designed to make six servings. Essential equipment to have to hand is a juicer, which you will need to make most of the breakfast drinks; you will also need a blender/liquidizer (hand held is fine) to create super-smooth soups and, of course, smoothies!

Juices and Smoothies

These vibrant, nutritious drinks are bursting with essential vitamins, minerals and other elements that will keep you going and ensure that your blood-sugar levels remain stable.

Carrot, apple & ginger juice

This zingy, colourful juice will provide the perfect start to your day. There's no need to peel the carrots or the apples – there is plenty of goodness in their skins!

  5 large carrots
  1 whole apple
  1cm piece of fresh root ginger, peeled

Pop all of the ingredients into your juicer together. Pour the resulting juice over ice, and sip slowly through a straw.

Celery, cucumber & spinach juice

Vegetable juices are a mainstay of the Drop Zone Diet and provide a wealth of key nutrients. This fresh, delicious juice is pumped full of vitamins and minerals that will keep you going for hours.

> 6 celery sticks
> 7.5cm piece of cucumber
> 100g fresh spinach, rinsed
> 1cm piece of fresh root ginger, peeled

Pop all of the ingredients into your juicer together. Pour the resulting juice over ice, and sip slowly through a straw.

Summer fruits juice

The best thing about this juice is that it can be prepared all year round, even when summer berries are out of season. Berries lose none of their goodness when they are frozen, and it's a good idea to keep some in the freezer for an emergency boost. This juice is a Drop Zone Diet favourite!

> juice of 2 oranges, freshly squeezed
> juice of ½ a lime, freshly squeezed
> 100ml still mineral water
> 150g frozen berries (blueberries, raspberries and strawberries are ideal, but anything will do)
> 4 ice cubes

Place all of the ingredients into a liquidizer and blend until smooth. Drink immediately.

Pepper, broccoli & ginger juice

This may sound like an odd combination, but the ginger lifts this nutritious juice to sublime heights! Broccoli is one of the most nutrient-rich vegetables around and has a fresh, subtle taste that makes it ideal for juices.

> 1 whole yellow pepper, including seeds and stem
> 300g fresh broccoli, including stalk
> 2 celery sticks
> 1cm piece of fresh root ginger, peeled

Pop all of the ingredients into your juicer together. Pour the resulting juice over ice, and sip slowly through a straw.

Avocado high-energy drink
This smooth, delicious drink is not only filling enough to act as a main meal, but it delivers a burst of essential fats to aid concentration and improve skin and hair.

> ½ small avocado, peeled and pitted
> 2 tablespoons low-fat plain live yoghurt
> 120ml still mineral water
> juice of ½ a lime, freshly squeezed
> juice of 1 orange, freshly squeezed

Place all of the ingredients into a liquidizer and blend until smooth. Drink immediately.

Orange & pomegranate juice
Both oranges and pomegranates are rich in vitamin C – one pomegranate has almost 40 per cent of the recommended daily vitamin C requirement for adults – and antioxidants that will boost health on all levels.

juice of 2 oranges, freshly squeezed
juice of 1 pomegranate, freshly pressed (go to www.
jeannettejackson.com for how to juice a pomegranate)
50ml still mineral water

Use a juicer to extract the juice from both the oranges and the pomegranates. Blend with the water and drink immediately.

Banana & honey delight

This warm, soothing drink will provide you with a sustained source of energy for the evening, and also help to encourage good, restful sleep. When you finish the Drop Zone Diet, you may find it becomes a regular night-time treat.

200ml skimmed milk
1 small banana, sliced
1 teaspoon Manuka honey
5 whole pecan nuts

Heat the milk in a small pan over a low heat until hot, but not boiling. While the milk is warming, grind or crush the nuts as finely as you can. Place your sliced banana, milk, honey and nuts into a liquidizer and blend until smooth. Drink immediately.

Celery, cucumber & ginger juice

This fresh, light juice has an almost instant impact upon bloating and water retention, and will help to alleviate that first-thing-in-the-morning puffiness. The ginger will kick-start your digestive system, too!

6 celery sticks
7.5cm piece of cucumber
1cm piece of fresh root ginger, peeled

Pop all of the ingredients into your juicer together. Pour the resulting juice over ice, and sip slowly through a straw.

Mango smoothie

Mangoes are literally teeming with vibrant nutrients that will boost your energy levels and affect your health on all levels. This is a filling, satisfying smoothie that you'll want to make long after you've finished the Drop Zone Diet.

½ mango, peeled, stoned and sliced
2 tablespoons low-fat, plain live yoghurt
juice of 1 orange, freshly squeezed
1 teaspoon Manuka honey

Place all of the ingredients into a liquidizer and blend until smooth. Drink immediately.

Watercress & carrot juice

With its high vitamin C content, watercress supports the immune system, and is a rich source of iron to provide energy and oxygenated blood. Its lovely, peppery taste will get you going in the morning!

80g fresh rinsed watercress, leaves and stems
4 large carrots, chopped
100ml still mineral water
juice of ½ a lemon, freshly squeezed

Place all of the ingredients into a liquidizer and blend until smooth. Drink immediately.

Beetroot, cucumber & ginger juice

Beetroot contains a natural chemical that reduces inflammation, allowing every cell and organ in the body to perform more efficiently. This radiant red drink will lift your mood and energy levels for the day to come.

  1 fresh beetroot, peeled and chopped into chunks
  ½ cucumber, chopped into chunks
  1cm piece of fresh root ginger, peeled

Place all of the ingredients into a juice machine and blend until smooth. Drink immediately.

Soups

Warm, nutritious soups form the backbone of the Drop Zone Diet. The following recipes will create enough for six 200ml servings. At some meals you will be adding rice cakes alongside. Don't eat more than two thin ones. At other meals you will be combining your soup with beans, such as adzuki or black-eyed beans. These add a little extra protein, and make your soup more filling. When they appear on the menu, simply warm 2 tablespoons of the beans suggested and when piping hot stir them into the soup. Tinned, drained beans are easiest; pop any leftovers into a sealed tub in your fridge and use as necessary throughout the diet. Eat slowly, to encourage healthy digestion.

Each soup will keep in the fridge for three days and in the freezer for three months. The recipes make more than is needed for the diet, so there is spare to freeze for when you have finished it.

Tomato, adzuki bean & chilli soup

A hint of chilli makes this nutritious, colourful soup even more warming and filing. The adzuki beans offer a good boost of protein, whilst the tomatoes are ready to work their antioxidant magic!

    450g fresh tomatoes, unpeeled
    ground white pepper and salt (to taste)
    3 cloves of garlic, unpeeled
    1 large onion, peeled and chopped
    100g leek, chopped
    20g celery, chopped
    ½ a medium red chilli (to taste)
    80g adzuki beans
    2 large tablespoons of tomato puree
    700ml water
    2 vegetable stock cubes
    2 tablespoons of red wine vinegar

Preheat the oven to 200°C/400°F/gas mark 6.

Slice the unpeeled tomatoes in half and place on a baking tray, sprinkle them with a generous amount of pepper and a touch of salt to taste, then place in the oven and bake for 30 minutes, adding the unpeeled garlic cloves after 25 minutes. Meanwhile, place the chopped onion, leek, celery and chilli in a heavy-bottomed saucepan with the adzuki beans and tomato puree, then cover with the 700ml of water. Add the 2 vegetable stock cubes and simmer for 20 minutes to allow the vegetables to soften. Remove the tomatoes and garlic from the oven, carefully peel the garlic, then add both to the pan, along with the red wine vinegar, and simmer for a further 10 minutes. Allow the soup to cool, then blend until smooth.

Serve a 200ml portion with each meal as directed and freeze the remainder in batches of 200ml as spare meals for future use.

Carrot and ginger soup with brown rice

This brightly coloured, nutritious soup is surprisingly filling and contains a host of digestion-enhancing ingredients, plus a range of crucial B vitamins from the brown rice, which are essential for transforming carbohydrates into glucose to give you energy.

> 1 large onion, peeled and chopped
> 100g leek, chopped
> 20g celery, chopped
> 350g carrots, unpeeled and chopped
> 3 cloves of garlic, unpeeled
> 50g easy cook brown rice
> 1,200ml of water
> 2 vegetable stock cubes
> 20g freshly grated ginger
> salt and pepper

Place the chopped onion, leek and celery in a large, heavy-bottomed saucepan, along with the chopped carrots, garlic and brown rice. Add the 1,200ml of water and 2 vegetable stock cubes, then bring to boil and simmer for 40 minutes (ensure the rice has gone soft – top up with a little water, if necessary). Now add the fresh ginger, a generous amount of pepper and a touch of salt and cook for a further 10 minutes. Allow the soup to cool, then blend until smooth.

Serve a 200ml portion with each meal as directed and freeze the remainder in batches of 200ml as spare meals for future use.

Butternut squash & cumin soup with toasted pumpkin seeds and black-eyed beans

This mild yet spicy soup is bursting with nutritious vegetables to comfort and feed your very core. The EFA-rich pumpkin seeds feed your brain and provide a lovely nutty flavour, while the black-eyed beans help to provide bulk and essential proteins.

450g butternut squash, peeled, seeds removed and flesh cut into chunks
1 teaspoon vegetable oil
1 teaspoon ground cumin
1 large onion, peeled and chopped
100g leek, chopped
20g celery, chopped
150g carrot, peeled and chopped
3 cloves of garlic, peeled
800ml of water
2 vegetable stock cubes
30g black-eyed beans
2 tablespoons pumpkin seeds
juice of ½ lemon, freshly squeezed
ground white pepper

Preheat the oven to 180°C/350°F/gas mark 4.

Place the butternut squash chunks in an ovenproof dish, then toss them in the vegetable oil and ground cumin. Place in the oven for about 25 minutes, until the squash is soft and just starting to go brown. Meanwhile, put the chopped onions, leeks, celery, carrots and garlic in a large pan. Cover with the 800ml of water and add the 2 vegetable stock cubes, then simmer for 20 minutes, allowing the vegetables to go soft. When ready, add the oven-roasted squash pieces and the black-eyed beans to the pan and cook for a further 10 minutes, adding more water, if necessary. Place a little oil in a frying pan and toast the pumpkin seeds until they turn slightly brown. Allow the soup to cool, add the toasted seeds, along with the juice of half a freshly squeezed lemon and season with white pepper, then blend until smooth.

Serve a 200ml portion with each meal as directed and freeze the remainder in batches of 200ml as spare meals for future use.

Spinach & nutmeg soup with quinoa and butter beans

This vibrant green soup is high in energy-giving iron and protein, and is lovely served both hot or cold. Spinach is a great source of beta-carotene, which is a precursor to vitamin A and essential for healthy skin. The quinoa, which is a grain, provides low-fat protein.

1 large onion, peeled and chopped
100g leek, chopped
20g celery, chopped
3 cloves of garlic, chopped
50g quinoa
700ml water
2 vegetable stock cubes
½ teaspoon of nutmeg, grated
40g tinned butter beans, drained and washed
100g baby spinach leaf

ground white pepper and salt
fresh lemon juice

Place the chopped onion, leek and celery in a large saucepan, along with the fresh garlic and quinoa. Add the 700ml of water and 2 vegetable stock cubes and bring to boil, then gently simmer for 20 minutes, allowing the vegetables to soften. Using a stick blender, blend in the grated nutmeg, the butter beans and spinach, and flavour with lots of white pepper and a pinch of salt. Put a lid on the pan and cook for a further 5 minutes. Allow the soup to cool, add the juice of half a fresh lime, then blend until smooth.

Serve a 200ml portion with each meal as directed and freeze the remainder in batches of 200ml as spare meals for future use.

Meals

The following recipes are finely balanced to offer key nutrients to keep hunger at bay, and to encourage good health on all levels. The portions may be small, but the meals are perfectly formed and an essential part of the Drop Zone Diet.

Banana Melt

Bananas are considered little packets of energy because of the wealth of nutrients they contain. One banana also contains 16 per cent of your daily fibre requirements, which will get your digestive system moving!

½ small banana, sliced
½ wholegrain pitta bread, toasted

2 walnuts, roughly chopped
1 teaspoon Manuka honey

Place the sliced banana (keep the other half of the banana in its skin and eat mid-morning as a snack) in the middle of your toasted pitta bread. Top with the chopped walnuts and drizzle with honey, then serve.

Pineapple & melon medley

This is a surprisingly filling breakfast that also provides you with a series of snacks to nibble throughout the morning, to keep your blood sugar and energy levels steady.

2 slices fresh pineapple, peeled and cored
2 slices cantaloupe melon, peeled and seeds removed
2 tablespoons low-fat, plain live yoghurt
1 teaspoon Manuka honey

Place half the fruit in a bowl and top with yoghurt and honey. The remaining fruit can be eaten throughout the morning.

Avocado & rice cakes

This may appear like a light lunch, but it's more filling than you'd think! Avocados are a great source of monounsaturated fats and protein to keep you going for hours.

½ large avocado, peeled, stoned and thinly sliced
3 thin rice cakes

Place the sliced avocado onto the rice cakes. Eat one avocado-topped rice cake every hour over a three-hour period (from noon to 2pm, for example, or whenever you take your lunch).

Lymph & liver tonic cleanse

Grapefruits are a traditional liver cleanser and lemon also works to encourage liver function. Mange tout and kale are rich in antioxidants and add a little crunch to keep you full for longer.

> juice of 2 large grapefruits, freshly squeezed
> 500ml still mineral water
> 60g mange tout
> 60g fresh kale
> juice of ½ a lemon, freshly squeezed

Blend together the grapefruit juice and water, and sip slowly over one hour. As you are doing so, lightly steam the vegetables until they are just tender, and squeeze over the lemon juice. Nibble on these throughout the afternoon or evening, chewing slowly.

Cod with green beans & courgettes

Cod is a great source of omega-3 fats and also a good, low-calorie form of protein. Lovely summer vegetables round out this tasty, satisfying meal.

> 100g cod fillet
> 50g green beans
> 1 courgette
> 1 teaspoon olive oil
> sea salt and freshly ground black pepper (to taste)
> juice of ½ a lemon, freshly squeezed

Preheat the oven to 180°C/350°F/gas mark 4.

Using a steamer basket, steam the cod over a pan of boiling water for about 10 minutes, then add the green beans and steam for a further 5 minutes.

As the cod is steaming, cut the courgette in half lengthways and brush both sides of each slice with a little olive oil. Season to taste with sea salt and black pepper, and then place on a baking tray in the preheated oven. Roast for 10 minutes, and then remove.

Place the cod, courgette and beans on a plate, season to taste, and squeeze over the lemon juice. Serve immediately.

Salmon with corn on the cob

Another fantastic source of omega-3 fats, salmon is a rich and satisfying source of protein that will keep you going all evening. These fats also help your brain to work better and improve your memory!

> 100g fresh salmon fillet
> 1 sweetcorn on the cob
> juice of ½ a lemon, freshly squeezed

Grill or pan-fry the salmon for about 7 minutes – it should still be a nice bright pink colour and moist inside. While it is cooking, steam the sweetcorn over a pot of boiling water for about 8 minutes, or until tender. Place the salmon and sweetcorn on a plate and squeeze over the lemon juice. Serve immediately.

Egg-white omelette with tomatoes, mushrooms & walnuts

This may seem like an unusual combination, but I guarantee you'll love it. It packs a big protein punch to provide you with steady energy levels throughout the evening.

3 small free-range eggs
sea salt and freshly ground black pepper (to taste)
4 medium flat mushrooms, washed and trimmed
1 medium tomato, halved
4 walnuts, roughly chopped

Separate two of the eggs and place the whites in a bowl. Add the final egg whole (white and yolk) to the egg whites and beat until smooth. Stir in a little sea salt and black pepper to taste.

Slice the tomatoes in half and grind over some sea salt and black pepper to taste. Place on a baking tray alongside the mushrooms and grill for approximately 10 minutes.

After 5 minutes pour the omelette mixture into a non-stick frying pan, spreading it evenly around the base, using a spatula to ensure the mixture stays even on the bottom of the pan. When the underside is done, after approximately 3 minutes, toss the omelette and cook the other side. When all the ingredients are cooked, place on a plate and scatter everything with the chopped walnuts.

Egg & prawns with fresh greens

This is a spectacularly quick and nutritious meal. You can boil your egg in advance and then assemble in just minutes. Prawns are rich in protein and energy-boosting B vitamins.

50g fresh spinach, washed
1 large free-range egg, hard-boiled, peeled and sliced
60g cooked prawns
¼ red pepper, diced
1 fresh beetroot, boiled or roasted and diced
juice of ½ a lemon, freshly squeezed

Place the spinach on a plate and arrange the egg, prawns, pepper and beetroot on top. Squeeze over the fresh lemon juice and serve.

Grilled turkey with tomatoes & mushrooms

It takes less than 20 minutes to prepare and cook this dish, and there will only be one pan to wash! Because it contains the soothing amino acid tryptophan, turkey will almost guarantee you a good night's sleep!

200g turkey escalope
1 medium tomato, halved
sea salt and freshly ground black pepper, to taste
6 small mushrooms, peeled and sliced
juice of ½ a lemon, freshly squeezed (optional)

Preheat the grill to high, and place the turkey escalope on a grill pan. Season the tomato and place alongside the turkey, then surround everything with the sliced mushrooms. Grill for approximately 10 minutes, turning the turkey halfway through cooking. Serve immediately with a squeeze of fresh lemon juice, if desired.

Prawn, asparagus & spinach salad

This salad makes a lovely evening meal or light lunch, both during and after you've finished the diet. Asparagus contains prebiotics, which stimulate the growth of friendly bacteria in the gut and encourage optimum digestion.

6 asparagus tips, washed
60g cooked prawns
100g fresh spinach, washed

6 cherry tomatoes, halved
juice of ½ a lemon, freshly squeezed

Steam the asparagus tips over a pan of boiling water for about 5 minutes, or until tender to the point of a knife. While they are cooking, arrange the spinach on a plate and scatter with the tomatoes. Arrange the prawns on top, add the cooked asparagus and squeeze over the lemon juice.

Vegetarian Options

Pineapple & cashew nut sweet rice

You can serve this rice either warm or cold, so if time is tight you may want to prepare it the night before. The flavour combination is simple, but hugely delicious!

50g easy-cook brown rice
250g tinned kidney beans, drained
30g pineapple slices, fresh or tinned
6 cashew nuts
soy sauce (optional)

Boil the rice according to the instructions on the packet (usually for about 10 to 12 minutes). While the rice is cooking, heat the kidney beans in a small saucepan. When the rice is cooked, drain well and then stir in the pineapple, kidney beans and cashew nuts. Add a dash of soy sauce, if desired, and serve immediately.

Warm lemon & lentil salad

You'll enjoy this delicious, fragrant salad whether you are a vegetarian or not! Top with a little black pepper, if desired, but give the salt a miss as the lentils will have absorbed plenty while in the tin.

> 1 red pepper, seeds removed and quartered
> 1 teaspoon olive oil
> 30g tinned puy lentils, drained
> 1 handful fresh watercress, leaves and stems, washed
> 1 tablespoon dried cranberries
> juice of ½ a lemon, freshly squeezed

Preheat the oven to 200°C/400°F/gas mark 6.

Brush the pepper quarters with olive oil, and roast in the preheated oven for approximately 20 minutes. While the peppers are cooking, heat the lentils in a small saucepan. Place the watercress on a plate, top with the warm lentils and roasted peppers, and sprinkle with the cranberries. Squeeze over the lemon juice and serve.

Baked mushrooms with pine nuts

Portobello mushrooms have a nice, meaty texture, making this meal surprisingly filling. They are also rich in B vitamins, which help to supply energy and reduce the impact of stress on your body.

> ¼ small onion, finely chopped
> 20g porridge oats
> 1 clove garlic, peeled and crushed
> 100g fresh tomatoes, chopped
> 20g pine nuts, chopped
> 2 large flat mushrooms (i.e., Portobello), washed
> juice of ½ a lemon, freshly squeezed
> 1 whole beef tomato, sliced, to serve

Preheat the oven to 180°C/350°F/gas mark 4.

In a small bowl, combine the onion, oats, garlic, tomatoes and pine nuts and mix together thoroughly. Put the mushrooms on a baking tray, and spoon the mixture into the cups of the mushrooms. Squeeze over the lemon juice. Roast in the preheated oven for 15 minutes. Serve with sliced tomato.

Healthy bean burrito

This is a quick and nourishing take on a traditional Mexican burrito. The little hit of chilli powder will warm and stimulate your digestion.

> 1 teaspoon olive oil
> 1 clove garlic, peeled and crushed
> ½ red onion, peeled and sliced
> ½ red pepper, seeds removed and diced
> 20g tinned black-eyed beans, drained
> 1 pinch chilli powder
> 1 wholewheat flour tortilla

Preheat the oven to 200°C/400°F/gas mark 6.

Blend together the olive oil and garlic. Place the onions and peppers in an ovenproof dish, and brush them with the garlic oil. Roast for 15 to 20 minutes, stirring occasionally. While the onions and peppers are cooking, warm the beans in a small saucepan and stir in the chilli powder. Remove the onions and peppers from the oven when cooked, and combine with the beans. Place the mixture in the centre of a wholewheat flour tortilla, and serve.

Minted three-bean salad

Like all pulses, beans are a magnificent source of vegetable protein, and very low in fat. Brightly coloured beans, such as kidney beans, are also rich in antioxidant nutrients – the anti-ageing ones!

> 1 tablespoon tinned kidney beans, drained
> 1 tablespoon tinned adzuki beans, drained
> 1 tablespoon tinned butter beans, drained
> 1 handful salad greens, washed and torn
> juice of ½ a lime, freshly squeezed
> 1 tablespoon white wine vinegar
> ½ tablespoon mint sauce

Place the mixed beans in a small saucepan and heat through. While they are warming, combine the lime juice, vinegar and mint sauce in a small bowl to make the dressing and set aside. Place the salad greens on your plate, top with the warmed beans, and pour over the dressing. Serve immediately.

Warm pumpkin & chickpea salad

The vibrant colours of this delicious dish are sure to tempt you. Rich in antioxidants and protein – and flavour – this is an ideal dish for vegetarians and carnivores alike!

> 25g fresh pumpkin, peeled, seeds removed and flesh cubed
> 2 teaspoons olive oil
> 1 clove of garlic, peeled and crushed
> 75g tinned chickpeas, drained
> 1 handful fresh spinach, washed
> ½ small onion, finely chopped

Preheat the oven to 180°C/350°F/gas mark 4.

In an ovenproof dish, toss the pumpkin in the olive oil and stir in the garlic. Roast in the preheated oven for about 20 minutes, until soft to the point of a knife. Just before the pumpkin is cooked, place the chickpeas in a small saucepan over a gentle heat until warm. Create a bed of spinach on a plate, top with the warm chickpeas and pumpkin, and sprinkle over the chopped onion. Serve immediately.

PART THREE
Day 15 and Beyond

The One Where We Make
the Most of Feeling Great

Congratulations! You've finished the Drop Zone Diet and I am confident that you are feeling better than you have in years! You weigh less and you are fitting into your old clothes you haven't worn in ages. Best of all, you are full of vigour and determination; you are sleeping better and waking up energized; your hair and skin are glowing with good health; and you've broken bad habits that have caused you to gain weight in the past. So what happens now?

It's time to make the most of your achievement. If you've lost the weight you wanted to lose, you'll have to tread carefully to ensure that you don't put it all back on again by reverting to your previous lifestyle. There are some simple ways to ensure that you remain at your new, lighter weight, and we'll look at these shortly. If you still have more weight to lose, you can embark upon the Drop Zone Diet again in three months' time. Until then, follow the instructions below for healthy weight maintenance and continue to make healthy choices when you are faced with temptation. Under no circumstances does your post-Drop Zone Diet lifestyle have to be extreme. There will always be times when you eat or drink a little more than you should, or give in to a takeaway or even a double-chocolate brownie sundae. The secret of long-term success is to be realistic. If your diet is 80 per cent healthy, then the other 20 per cent simply doesn't matter so much. Try to remember that succumbing to a treat (or more than one) doesn't mean you've 'wrecked' your diet or your new approach to food. It simply means that you'll need to be a little firmer with yourself tomorrow and maybe even the next day, and you'll need to remind yourself why this new, healthy lifestyle is right for you. A look in the mirror will confirm the reasons!

Doing the Maths

After the simplicity of the Drop Zone Diet, the last thing you'll want to do is to start counting calories, but it does help with weight maintenance to be aware of the figures. In general, it takes roughly 3,500 calories to create an extra pound of fat. One pound may not seem like a lot, but they can add up pretty quickly and you could find yourself back where you started before you know it. For example, if you had a large mocha coffee every day on the way to work and a couple of extra potatoes with your dinner, you'll be taking in 500 extra calories. Over the course of a week, you've gained a pound without even noticing. Calories all add up – and accumulate on your hips, tummy and thighs!

It also makes sense that if you do want to eat a little more, you'll have to up the exercise. Once again, the maths is the same: by burning off 3,500 calories you'll lose a pound. So if you are planning to spend an afternoon sampling the delights of your local patisserie, you can probably counterbalance it by walking all the way home – at speed! Obviously you don't have to be that extreme, but it's worth remembering that being more active will compensate for periods when you are overeating. Some women find that they are naturally hungrier in the run-up to their periods, and experience more cravings during this time. Not only can you use my handy list of alternatives to typical food cravings (see pages 61–2), but you can book in an extra class at the gym, walk to the station instead of getting the bus, or even just take a good brisk walk after dinner every evening to keep things moving. To help you make some calculations, you may like to know that, on average, an hour of brisk walking burns about 400 calories, an hour of dancing burns about 500 calories and an hour of swimming closer to 600 calories. (If you only manage 20 minutes of any of these forms of exercise, then cut the figure by a third.)

Fat Sticks!

Food should be delicious, nutritious rocket-fuel for your body and help to keep you working at the optimum level. If you shift your mindset so that you begin to choose food according to its ability to make you healthy and well, rather than just stuffing it in because it looks nice or you feel tempted, you'll be making a good start. We often eat not because we are hungry but because we want to change the way we feel. The truth is that a sugary, fatty treat may make you feel better in the short term, but the consequences of that type of 'feeding' stick! Fat sticks not only to your thighs, stomach and buttocks, but to your self-esteem and confidence, too. Most of us feel guilt when we give in to temptation, which lowers our self-esteem and self-belief, and that's one sure way to start gaining weight again. Believe in your ability to make the right choices. Think about why you want to eat a particular food and see if you can come up with a healthier alternative – or do without it altogether. If you are having a rubbish day, why not benefit from those amazing endorphins that exercise creates? It's a sure way to lift your mood quickly and efficiently, and there will be no guilt involved.

Before you eat anything, ask yourself this critical question: 'Am I really hungry or do I simply want to alter my mood?' If it's the latter, look for non-food alternative.

Develop Some Strategies

It isn't always easy to stick to a plan – even one that benefits you so tremendously – so it helps to have some ammunition as back-up if you do end up in a battle with food.

• If you want to change the way you feel, refer back to pages 57–60 and take a look at the Positive Health Action column. Work out what action you could take that would create a shift in your energy. Book a class, join a group, visit a friend or busy yourself in a project that will engage you. Actions like these really work to create a mental shift.

• Remind yourself that you can control your brain. You may have to go back and retrain your RAS (see page 102) or your executive brain (see pages 104–5) and establish some new goals, but it's worth doing. Even simply reminding yourself of your existing goals can make a difference. Getting your brain in gear and on your side will make everything much easier.

• If you are genuinely hungry, then go with it for a while. Set yourself mini goals, for example, 'I'll see how I feel in 15 minutes'. If you're still thinking of food after 15 minutes, have a glass of hot water with the juice of half a lemon and a little honey, which will take the edge off things.

• Remember that the supplements are there to support you; take these for 14 days following the diet, and longer if necessary. Many people who have blood-sugar issues benefit from taking chromium in the long term (see page 123).

• Think about someone whose lifestyle (and figure or appearance) you admire. What do you think he or she would do in this situation? Successful people leave clues. Copy them; see them in your mind's eye and try them out for yourself.

• Unlearning old habits is a crucial part of your long-term success, and this can take some time, particularly if you aren't concentrating on making and sustaining changes. It takes an average of 21 days for new behaviour to become a habit, and the Drop Zone Diet lasts just 14 days. You may have a little more work to do to turn your bad habits into good ones.

• Remember that feeling slightly hungry is OK – and it's probably a better feeling than being stuffed to the gills and unable to move! Try to get used to that 'lighter' experience.

• If you do decide to succumb to something unhealthy, make sure you enjoy it and don't beat yourself up afterwards! Confirm to yourself that you have made the decision in your executive brain, and that it was an adult decision. Taking responsibility for our actions empowers us and helps us to develop a greater awareness of how and why we act the way we do. This enables us to make positive long-term changes in the future.

• Food should never be a battleground, so if this is the case, then why not book an appointment with a hypnotherapist or counsellor and try to work out how your relationship with food developed. This is a great way to learn some alternative coping strategies that will work for you as an individual.

• Lastly, how about going to night school and learning about nutrition? There are some fantastic local classes where you can learn the basics; who knows, it might become a brand-new career for you!

The Post-Drop-Zone-Diet Diet!

Losing all that weight so quickly will hopefully have made you very determined to keep it off and perhaps to even lose more. The first thing you need to do is make sure that you don't immediately return to your old habits. For the next 14 days, I suggest that you continue to eat the Drop Zone Diet soups as a main meal at least once a day. Not only will you benefit from their health-giving nutrients, but you'll also have at least one fairly low-calorie meal per day without experiencing any hunger pangs or cravings. The breakfast juices and smoothies are also a fabulous way to start your day. I hope it will become second nature to prepare a healthy breakfast for yourself, and these drinks are undoubtedly the quickest, most efficient way to get a healthy dose of nutrients (not to mention energy) with the minimum of fuss.

The truth is that good-quality, healthy food is not fattening. If you base your diet around a few key principles, and watch your portion sizes, you will not gain weight. For the record, portion sizes do matter. Remember the example of the bottomless soup bowls (see page 104). If there's food on your plate, you'll probably eat it. Go small at the outset; you can always eat more if you are hungry later on. If you fill your plate every night, choose a smaller plate! If you eat mindfully, thinking about what you are eating and concentrating on the act, you are more likely to hear the messages from your old friends the hormones leptin and grehlin (see page 90), who will tell you when you are full.

Foods to include

Fruit and vegetables
As many as you can manage and as brightly coloured and varied as possible. The Drop Zone Diet contains a veritable rainbow of fruit and vegetables, and the key nutrients they provide will keep your body healthy and help to eliminate cravings. The vast majority are also low in calories, so you can get used to filling up your plate without tipping the scales. Potatoes can be included after you've finished the Drop Zone Diet but eat them sparingly. Although they are vegetables, they are also carbs, which should be eaten as part of a balanced diet. We all tend to eat too many spuds, just to bump up the meal. Two-thirds of a small potato, a few times a week, can help to fill you up and provide a great source of fibre if you keep the skin on.

Whole grains

Whole grains mean that nothing has been stripped or removed from the grains; they are not refined. So wholemeal bread is a whole grain, while white bread is not – the refining process changes it from being 'whole'. Whole grains offer a complete package of nutrients that is perfectly balanced – rich in vitamins E and B, a little protein, some iron, and a host of minerals such as magnesium and selenium, and lots of fibre. The best sources are barley, oats, buckwheat, corn, millet, quinoa, brown and wild rice, rye and wheat. I don't recommend that you eat pasta or bread for the first month after you finish the Drop Zone Diet, but you can include other grains – adding them to your delicious soups, or underneath a lovely piece of grilled fish or roasted vegetables. If you aren't convinced, remember that whole grains offer sustained energy and limit the risk of insulin resistance (see page 67).

Fish and shellfish

Aim for two or three servings a week to benefit from the healthy EFAs they contain. Most fish provides good-quality protein with comparatively few calories, providing you steam or grill it rather than fry it in batter or slather it with sauce! The nutrients contained in fish and shellfish will improve your mood, your brain function and your skin, hair and nails!

Dairy produce and eggs

Skimmed milk has just as much calcium and nutritional value as semi-skimmed or full-fat milk, so choose this for your tea or coffee or whole-grain breakfast cereal. Aim to include at least a few tablespoons of low-fat, plain live yoghurt in your diet every day to experience the benefits of the probiotics it contains. It will encourage healthy digestion and elimination, which means that your body will better utilize the nutrients you feed it. There is nothing wrong with cheese – everything in moderation – but it's easy to get carried away. Learn to grate and sprinkle rather than cut or even 'chunk'. A piece of cheese the size of your thumb will offer a nice dose of calcium and satisfy you, particularly if it's grated, which makes it go that much further. Similarly, butter is a nutritious part of a healthy diet *in moderation*. One pat of butter would ideally be enough to see you through a whole day. Always choose good-quality cheese and dairy produce.

Beans and pulses

These can form the basis of a healthy diet by providing an excellent source of complex (meaning slow-release, or unrefined) carbohydrates, which will provide you with energy. They'll also offer fibre, protein and key vitamins and minerals. They are low fat and an inexpensive addition to any diet. Many also contain iron, which can help to keep you feeling energized. Chickpeas, lentils, black-eyed beans, adzuki beans, kidney beans and borlotti beans are great choices, and you can eat them on their own or add them to salads, Drop Zone Diet soups and stews.

Nuts and seeds

These are great sources of EFAs and protein, and have a host of other health benefits as well (see page 146, for example). The secret is to have no more than four or five and then *put the bag away*. Always choose unsalted, raw nuts; the roasted ones tend to have oils added to them, which bumps up the calorie count.

Lean meat and poultry

Unless you are a vegetarian, these will probably form a fairly staple part of your diet. Good sources of protein and iron, meat and poultry can be eaten two or three times a week. The secret is in calculating the portion size. If it fits in the palm of your hand, it's about right. Try to be creative about your cooking methods. Stir-frying a pile of vegetables in a non-stick pan is obviously going to be far less calorific than frying them in oil.

Controlling caffeine

You've probably now become accustomed to getting by on one small skinny latte or a cup of regular tea each day, and doing without cola altogether. Why not continue with the regime? While a little caffeine can be stimulating, too much coffee or tea messes with your adrenal glands (the stress-hormone producers) and can leave you exhausted, no matter how well you are eating. And although caffeinated fizzy diet drinks may not contain calories, they don't contain any nutrients, either, and the new, slimmer, healthier you only puts food in your mouth that does something positive for your health. When giving up caffeine drinks, do ensure that you drink enough fluid throughout the day, as dehydration can cause you to become tired and cause cravings for food that will give you a quick, sugary boost of energy.

Foods to avoid

This list is much shorter but, dare I say it, probably includes most things you ate before you started the Drop Zone Diet. To have continued success, just flip your old eating routine on its head. You already know why you need to give most of these foods a miss: 'If you always do what you've always done, you'll always get what you've always got!' They add little if any nutritional value to your overall diet and they may even undermine it. None of these foods has featured in the Drop Zone Diet, and for good reason. Think about how well you've been feeling these past two weeks. If you re-introduce these foods *at any point*, you'll be much more likely to put on weight, feel more sluggish and experience cravings.

Processed or refined foods of any description

Go fresh and natural. Continue to try to cook your own meals from scratch; you'll truly benefit from the extra nutrients your body receives. Get into the habit of batch-cooking and freezing healthy soups and stews, and filling your fridge with nutritious snacks such as those you ate while on the Drop Zone Diet. Cakes, biscuits, crisps, processed meats, ready meals, white pasta and bread (see box, below), sugary cereals and white rice should come off the menu entirely.

Bread and pasta

Although whole-grain breads and pastas are healthy, it's a good idea to leave them off the menu for a month or so after finishing the diet. The reason for this is that they are heavy-duty carbohydrates that can play havoc with your newly balanced blood-sugar levels. I believe we eat too much bread and pasta in this country and the reason for this is not just habit but because it is readily available, quick and very easy, which appeals to our lazy side! Many people have toast for breakfast, a sandwich for lunch and pasta for dinner. It's refined-carb overload and it can be a massive strain on your digestive system. It's also far too easy to accompany them with high-fat sauces or spreads, many of which contain hidden sugars and salt that affect the fluid balance in your body and encourage water retention, so you look puffy and bloated again. So whilst white bread and pasta are out entirely, keep the whole-grain versions off the menu for the first month and then limit yourself to three or four portions a week, substituting healthy, colourful salads with quality lean protein and beans or whole grains in the interim.

Once digested, a single slice of white bread is converted into the same amount of glucose as four tablespoons of sugar.

Alcohol

Kate Moss once famously stated that nothing tastes as good as skinny feels. I know that right now you feel better than you have for ages. It's great to slip on those old jeans from years ago, and have room to move in them! So, if you want to keep the weight off, you have to cut down your alcohol intake. By now you are probably used to getting through the day without a tipple – and you may not even have noticed its absence. Try to maintain the same mindset. The more you drink, the more likely you are to put on weight – particularly around your waist – and the less efficiently your body burns fat and metabolizes the food you eat. I suggest continuing to abstain for 14 days after the Drop Zone Diet has finished, to allow the process of healing to continue and to get your metabolism back on track. After that, moderation is the key. You know how much is too much – and you also know how much you want to remain slim. It's a simple choice.

Condiments

The vast majority of condiments contain high levels of fats and sugars, not to mention other chemicals. Steer clear of them when you can. Use fresh lemon juice, vinegar, herbs, spices, a little soy sauce, sea salt and freshly ground black or white pepper to season your food and bring out the flavour. The good news is that you've developed a much finer palate on the Drop Zone Diet and probably appreciate the fresh, natural taste of good, healthy food much more than in the past. There's no need to mask it with junk! You'll be adding unnecessary calories and undermining your retrained taste buds.

Sugar

We have talked at length about why sugar needs to be removed from your diet on a permanent basis. There are a number of ways to eliminate sugar (see below) and I highly recommend that you use them. Avoid table sugar in any form, and all foods that contain refined sugar in its many guises. If you choose fresh, natural foods in their whole form, you'll benefit from the healthy, slow-release sugars they contain and won't even miss their nasty cousin, sucrose!

Eliminating sugar

- Drink herbal teas with lemon or honey instead of regular tea with white sugar

- Snack on fruit, which will satisfy sweet cravings, offer key nutrients and help to keep your blood-sugar levels more stable

- Eat regular meals to avoid afternoon sugar dips

- Try to eliminate stress to reduce the desire for evening munchies

- Avoid diet soft drinks, which can actually trick your body into thinking it's having something sugary, leaving you wanting more and more

- Eat a diet high in natural whole foods

And Finally . . .

Enjoy feeling more energized and vigorous. Make use of this energy to become more active, which not only burns calories and creates fat-burning muscle, but also improves your circulation, which impacts on every single organ in your body. Fitting in exercise even two or three times a week, for 15 minutes a time, will make a dramatic difference to your overall health and wellbeing, including reducing stress levels naturally, and will be one of the best tools you have to keep your weight in check.

Enjoy your food. You've been introduced to a whole new world of flavours and food combinations that have left you feeling vibrant and alive; what's more, you've seen how the pounds have dropped off and I'm sure you want more of the same! Experiment with food: have fun cooking new recipes and trying out new flavour combinations, herbs, spices and ingredients. Pick up fruit and vegetables you've never tried before and incorporate them into your diet. You don't have to eat a lot to enjoy good food, but enjoy it you should! If you are emotionally satisfied by your diet you are much more likely to be physically satisfied, too.

Above all, continue to believe in yourself and your goals. You've just proved that you can achieve results when you put your mind to it, and you can hold on to that realization and apply it to other areas of your life as well. Your new sense of confidence is attractive and inspirational and will motivate you to continue down the route of healthy living for years to come. And with healthy living comes balanced weight, abundant health and both inner and outer beauty.

Congratulations! You've made it this far and you are now on the path you want to continue down. If you have more weight to lose, you'll see it come off faster than you ever thought possible by sticking to the fundamental principles of the Drop Zone Diet. There is no need to continue with extreme eating for now (although you may enjoy another boosting stint of the 14-day diet plan in a few months time); instead, focus on what you've learned about eating well – how fresh, nutritious, whole foods can make you feel fantastic, remove those niggling cravings, encourage restful sleep and fill you with energy. You are looking better than ever and that will inspire you to go forward with confidence. If you design your meals around the principles above, you will succeed, no doubt.

The Drop Zone Diet creates a shift that is much bigger than weight loss. Many people 'find' themselves again, and remember the person they once were before they hid in baggy clothes, declined invitations and wore the same old outfits over and over again because they couldn't face the changing-room mirrors. The transformation is often so great, and confidence so enhanced, that people change careers and lifestyles (one of my clients, at the age of 52, packed in her job and went trekking around Thailand).

You too can experience such a transformation on the Drop Zone Diet. It's a step towards a more colourful, fulfilled life. Relish it. Savour the essence of it, and then relax and bask in the delights it brings you.

I wish you all the love and luck in the world.

Resources

page 19   Hall, Martin Robert, *Optimize Yourself*

page 33   Covey, Stephen R., *7 Habits of Highly Effective People*

page 49   Carey, Nessa, *The Epigenetics Revolution*

page 50   Subhani, M. I. and Osman, Amber, 'The Human Mind is a Tabula Rasa' (Iqra University Research centre)

page 53   Suter, Dr Catherine, Li, C. C. Y., Cropley, J. E., Cowley, M. J., Preiss, T., Martin, D. I. K, et al, 'A Sustained Dietary Change Increases Epigenetic Variation in Isogenic Mice'

page 65   Hoebel, Dr John, 'Is Sugar Addictive'

page 66   DesMaisons, Dr Kathleen, *Potatoes Not Prozac*

page 68   Noordam, Raymond, Gunn, David A., Tomlin, Cyrena C., Maier, Andrea B. and Mooijaart, Simon P., et al, 'High Serum Glucose levels Associated with Higher Perceived Age'

page 69   Herrear, Blanca M. and Lindgren, Cecilia M., et al, 'The Genetics of Obesity'

page 74   Feinman, Lawrence and Leiber, Charles, 'Ethanol & Lipid Metabolism', *American Journal of Clinical Nutrition*

page 77   Guiliano, Mireille, *French Women Don't Get Fat*

page 79   McTamney, Paul (courtesy of), Alcohol Quiz, *www.StopDrinkingAlcohol.com*

page 85   Everson C. A., Bergmann, B. M., Rechtschaffen, A., 'Sleep Deprivation in the Rat: III. Total Sleep Deprivation'

page 86   Weil, Andrew and Gurgevich, Steven, *Heal Yourself with Medical Hypnosis*

page 89   McKenna, Paul, *I Can Make You Thin*

page 104   Wansink, Brian, Painter, James E., North, Jill, 'Bottomless Bowls: Why Visual Cues of Portion Size May Influence Intake'

Acknowledgements

This book is dedicated to my beautiful daughter Sarah, who has blessed my life with joy and love since the moment she came into the world almost twenty-one years ago. To my mum, Eileen: thank you for giving me the confidence to always follow my dreams, I love you. To Karen, my beautiful, wise sister: 'Somewhere Over The Rainbow', you and Mum both got me through my finals with tears, tissues and lots of giggles! There would be no scientist Jackson without you both encouraging and loving me every step of the way. To Darren, Alycia and Charlotte: thanks for all the sunshine giggles in Florida. To Jo, Doogie, Thomas and Isaac: where would I be without all the cuddles! To Roy, my dad: I miss you every day and pray for you. To Gabriel: who could have known we were so close to this for all those years? And now we're loving it! A HUGE thank you to all my beautiful friends: you helped me to stand tall and stay proud throughout the years; where would I ever be without you all. Big thanks to chef *extraordinaire* Oliver Thomas, for designing the soups with me.

A special thank you to Katy Follain at Michael Joseph for the amazing opportunity to write this book. To my editor Gill Paul and all the team at Penguin Books: thank you for your encouragement, your support and your faith. It meant such a lot to me as a newbie!

And last but not least, to every single person who came to see me as a private client or on one of my seminars. I learned so much from all of you: your strength, your tenacity and your quest to be healthy and well, that you inspired me and we learned together. Without you, this book would not exist, and I thank you from the bottom of my heart.

Onwards and upwards then, until the next time we meet

With love

Jeannette